RITUAL

&

HEALING

STORIES OF ORDINARY AND EXTRAORDINARY TRANSFORMATION

COLLECTED BY DON EULERT, PHD

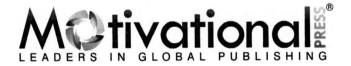

LEADERS IN GLOBAL PUBLISHING

Published by Motivational Press, Inc.
2360 Corporate Circle
Suite 400
Henderson, NV 89074
www.MotivationalPress.com

Manufactured in the United States of America.

ISBN: 978-1-62865-026-6

Contents

TRANSFORMATIVE EXPERIENCES WITH RITUAL

HEALING RITUALS IN PRACTICE

ACKNOWLEDGEMENTS

This book belongs to the contributing story-tellers, most of them first-time authors taking the risk of sharing personal experiences. Whether describing transformative events or daily attention to practices, they remind us that we are our stories, They encourage our own. Together these real-life stories are healing in themselves. Thank you also for your patience!

Thank you Monika Wikman and Vidya McNeill for envisioning and encouraging this book's beginnings, and Jessica Killebrew for your zealous reading of all the submissions and creating the first draft.

Appreciations to many others who believed and helped, who solicited friends and colleagues for contributions. In the seven years since this collection began, your encouragement and your excitement over the stories kept it alive.

With gratitude I think of the community who surrounded me with their warmth after the Witch fire, who immediately pitched in to rebuild our kiva, and who continue to bring ritual to life in our seasonal gatherings. We all give a hug to my son John Colby who prepares everything in the right way. In my thanks for your "tending the fireplace," I include all that you do for FrogFarm place and my time.

Gratitudes to Victoria Nicolosi and Amy Roost, for your enthusiasm for the project and for smiling through all those details of putting the collection into form and submission. You deserve co-editing credit.

To my partner Ute Jamrozy, who helped grow this book from the excitement of ideas we generated and shared around the firepit. I treasure our times together in preparation for solstice ceremonies, re-learning intentionality, paying attention, giving form to ideas about ritual. In bringing all together for the book, thank you for your patience, participation, love, and keen advice.

You all made this book happen; couldn't have done it without you!

INTRODUCTORY NOTE TO THE READER:
The Lost and Found

"I have come to suspect that in the absence of ritual, the soul runs out of its real nourishment,"   ***Malidoma Somé***

OR, TO PUT IT ANOTHER WAY, THE LOSS OF RITUAL LEAVES A HOLE IN THE heart of persons and society. In the place of solemn or celebratory markers of significance, our culture's iconic enactment is the disneyfied Super Bowl. Gang initiations replace rites of passage celebrated in community.

In my *Ritual and Healing* seminars and workshops over many years, I observe an increasing thirst for means of renewal and meaning-making. For years I envisioned an accessible and alive book on the topic. Maybe a summary from my seminars? *Not that interesting.* Maybe preach about lame rites of passage in our culture? Link the healing professions to the robes they have inherited from high priests and shamans?

Finally what excited this collection was to invite *"everybody's"* stories of ordinary and extraordinary experience with ritual, then see how they organize. The call for chapters asked the authors to explore how ritual attends a significant shift in meaning and perception in their life story. We asked,

In first-person narrative, describe an experience arising from ritual. The ritual setting may be a particular event or a longer practice that made " internal difference, / Where the Meanings, are . . ." for transformation and for psychological/physical healing.

This collection of real-life stories intends to encourage readers about the accessibility of ritual for their own lives and practice.

The stories in reply are amazing in depth, span, and authenticity, from Nevada's Burning Man festival to Albanian mourning rituals. Just now I finished reading through everything before writing this introduction, and I'm astonished. The authors' experience with ritual in their own lives and practice are poignant about what's lost and found; they provide access and encouragement.

From the sacred to the secular, the stories also define ritual (rite, ceremony) and purposes with such richness that little on that account needs be said here. Metzner's chapter reviews contemporary ritual behaviors; Krippner's preface describes the types historically. He also provides a succinct definition of the more formal/sacred performance:

definition "ritual"... *a prescribed, stylized, step-by-step, goal-directed performance of a mythological theme. It is "prescribed" by such practitioners as shamans, religious functionaries, or family or community elders.*

The Oxford dictionary definition from the Latin *ritus* (religious) also stresses the "solemn" and sacred, but then goes on to note "social and psychological" convention, "the habitual." That brings up the question I'm often asked: What's the difference between ritual and the habitual?

Metzner's description helps define:

Ritual is the purposive, conscious arrangement of a sequence of actions, at particular times and in particular places, according to specific intentions.

The habitual and routine (dinnertime, for example) might become ritualized by "conscious arrangement" and intention, as the Lawsons' chapter describes. With purpose and specific intentions, Elva Beach ritualizes cleaning her house. The ordinary can manifest significance, given attention and awareness. Every day we re-enact "generational wisdoms" simply through our physical being and actions. Ritualized or not, our choice. We are standing in the place of those gone before us. Now it's our turn, and responsibility, to be amazed at sunrise, a star-filled sky (or traffic). Interesting that both Cappadonna and Howell coin the term "Re-Membering" in the titles of their chapters.

Another question, "What's ritual for?" came up at a backyard barbeque (which has its own ritual overtones) last week. I reflect that she might have been asking "what's ritual good for anyway?" or, as a psychologist, "what psychological functions are served in ritual performance?"

Actually that's one question. From several chapters, a simple answer would be that we are made to feel safe. I imagine how, at the dawn of consciousness, primordial people created rituals to create a predictable order out of chaos, to protect the ego against disintegration.

The unexpected range of "functions served" as experienced by these writers is remarkable in what they let go (anger, grief, innocence) and find. What they find is personal, but here's a generalization. When ritual attention is paid, something creative happens. Ritual:

- Provides meaning, order, purpose, relationship.
- Helps with life-stage passages, transformation.
- Gives solidarity to cultural world-view and membership.
- Brings into life those things in our unconscious we do not ordinarily access.
- Re-minds that we belong to a supra-rational field of biological, cultural, psychological, and cosmological relationships.

"What's healed?" by *the purposive, conscious arrangement of a sequence of actions, at particular times and in particular places, according to specific intentions?* Biologically, with a change in our attitude, our "molecules of emotion" can do wonders. But in sum, most healing rituals intend the restoration of harmony, balance and relationship; then the rest will take care of itself. Navajo healing ceremonies, for example, locate the one to be healed (balanced) at various places in a depicted world of wholeness. Like the Tibetan prayer mandala, Navajo sand paintings in a healing ceremony are two-dimensional representations of a three-dimensional environment and multi-dimensional cosmology. Incantatory prayers call in powers from all the directions for the one to be healed.

When I woke up afterward, I never thought that my fall off the roof onto the rocks below was going kill me. "Hospital staph" was now another consideration. From trauma hospital to the insuranced placement, nobody paid much attention to the tube that emergency stuck through my back ribs to drain a collapsed lung.

After awhile this staph infection, seemingly immune to antibiotics, comes to the attention of the chief surgeon. I notice the epilates on his hospital garb for daily rounds. He seems impatient to perform the inevitable. Every day he describes how he will do the lung cavity surgery. Split the rib cage and fold back. By this time the infection will be crystallized, so he'll need to scrape the lungs before swabbing them down, and then good luck with that.

Friends notice this nocebo (opposite of the positive placebo) effect taking me down. They arrange a healing ceremony in my hospital room, under the direction of Dr. Coyote (we'll call him). He's an M.D. friend who spent years of learning and practice in the Navajo Nation.

He asks that friends and family in the bedside circle bring a talisman object, imbued with their healing intentions, for an altar. Dr. Coyote circles up and smudges for performance of ritual attention and intentional outcome. Then here comes the surgeon. After an exchange that established that Coyote knows medical-speak, surgeon backs out, with a "Well, good luck with *that*" attitude. Then everybody spoke and then Coyote invoked powers of the six directions. Everything got prayed for, including the wheezing suction machine and the rose color in the tube from my lung, not to get cloudy. Lifted by Ken's flute playing, I drifted over to the red rock canyons east of Gallup. All was as should be; beauty surrounds us. The ritual's attitude adjustment charged everybody in the circle, and was the beginning of my recovery—with no surgery.

The call for "all my relations" in healing rituals also includes restoring relationship with our own unattended fears or gratitudes, healing our separation from the underworld parts of the psyche. (Readers can journey there in chapters by Plotkin, Davis, Lukoff, Fleuridas, among others). The symbols, motifs, and patterns of ritual resonate with the archetypal. C.G. Jung even suggests that when we're in distress, a corresponding archetype is called up and "brings about a spiritual preparation" in the form of "magical ceremonies, sacrifices, invocations, prayers, and suchlike" (*CW* V, p. 294).

The restoration of relationship may be social, cultural, psychological, cosmological, or all of the above. My friend Jack from the Institute told me that Jung witnessed elders at the top of Taos Pueblo whose job it was to make the sun come up for everybody. Emptying lungs into their hands, at the right moment they threw the breath of life into the void, praying for life's renewal. In return, the sunrise! Beyond cause and effect, In this symbolic function not a day could go by without the pueblo's active relationship with the source of life.

That something needs to be sacrificed for renewal seems an archetypal pattern. Surely that's inherent in our psychological development as we leave one stage of life behind and move to the next (attended by rites of passage, one hopes). But this knowledge of sacrifice necessary for new life, inherent in our psychology and in nature, can be misconstrued and made literal. The Aztecs and Mayans are not the only cultures manifesting blood sacrifice. It's rooted in mythologies Norse to Egyptian, in religions pre-Christian and Christian. And in ritual abuse. Scarification and genital mutilation come to mind. As Metzner emphasizes, ritual itself (with its structured elements) is neutral.

And at best, an element of sacrifice or suffering, at least some physical engagement, seems important in full-blown rituals of transformation and rites of passage. To get out of ordinary space and time we need to get out of our heads. Wes Chester preoccupies juvenile delinquents with power tools. Several writers describe wilderness rites of passage, vision-quest fasting, participation in indigenous ceremonies—Beck in a sweat lodge, Hescamilla in the grave for an overnight of attention. Whether self-inflicted or in strict religious practice, deprivation (a sacrifice, cousin of suffering) often comes up as necessary to obtain clarity of vision, even access to the sacred.

About ritual and the sacred, I'll follow up on the earlier mention (the Oxford definition of ritual rooted in the religious, the "solemn and sacred"). Many of the chapters incorporate orthodox religious faith. More of them find the sacred in nature, and some "make" the sacred through ritual. Is the sacred something to be *found* (in nature or a deity), so that we can ritually go there and bring it back? Or do we *make* the sacred? -- ritualize a stone wall, a flag, a sunrise, a pilgrimage destination, a relationship-- so that when we go there we can participate in the sacred also. Perhaps the numinosity of the sacred locates in our collective unconscious, waits for the tools of ritual process to bring to the light of consciousness this inherent human trait.

If you want to go further into these mysteries, I recommend Mircea Eliade's ***The Sacred and the Profane***. He suggests that sacred ritual collapses time so that we not only enact but participate in our beginnings, in an "eternal return." To him, the sacred contains all reality/value. Other things contain reality to the extent that they participate in the sacred.

Now back to the beginnings of this Introduction, about the lost and found of ritual in our society. Perhaps everyone in our informational age (whose time is linear and goes off into the future), perhaps everyone still carries nostalgia for the loss of significant rituals. Our clocks are set to the cycle of seasonal markers. Waiting for rain, waiting out long nights for the return of light, would be life-long and primary in ritual attention to a hunter-gatherer or an agrarian culture. Postmodern we, with a flick, make light and heat or switch our identities. For better or worse, some things are lost.

Not that ritual will ever go away. These writers describe the plural emergences that fit to our era. And in our times still each person's childhood has a story-line punctuated with symbolism and ceremony, ritual elements (including suffering) and community recognition. We each remember significant "emergences" on our path toward adolescence. But as the last two chapters describe, without community-recognized rites of passage we have 30-year-old adolescents and youth "at risk" *and all kinds of social problems then ensue.*

My own growing up "country" was a pre-modern, even tribal, culture. Always at the mercy of weather and seasons, regular mealtimes with food we raised and prayed over. Chores. A one-room country school that was also the community center for seasonal "programs" in which every kid performed, and everybody-- even the bachelor farmers-- attended and applauded. Every Fall a time to ready crop and livestock to show and be judged at the Russell County Fair (and, the carnival!). Church on Sunday, catechism on Saturday, where I most sincerely studied "The Office of Keys and Confession" as passage to the sacred. This path through adolescence a matter of following things in their right order-- calving, weaning, and butchering; planting and harvesting. I was privileged to have been embedded in those natural cycles and in community, that reference.

But as with all our various childhood markers, they are lost. Now we all are left to find significance and renewals through *intentional acts concerning vital, existential human concerns* (Krippner). That's the *why* of ritual. Each person's ordinary and extraordinary healing story in this collection describes the *how.*

I hope that you the reader enjoy the variety and depth of these experiences shared. I hope you will be encouraged to find (or more appreciate your practice of) ritual to enrich you own life with psychological and physical healing. Pass it on . . . especially to teenagers.

Share your story at www.ritualandhealing.com

Good Road! Don Eulert

FORWARD
We Still Need Rituals
In The Twenty-First Century

STANLEY KRIPPNER, PhD,
SAYBROOK UNIVERSITY, SAN FRANCISCO,
CALIFORNIA

RITUALS CAN BE DEFINED AS STEP-BY-STEP PROCEDURES INTENDED TO ATTAIN a specified goal. However, the "steps" in the process generally occur in a fixed order and this order can be discerned by shifts in activity, gestures, songs, words, or other behaviors. Among indigenous people, most rituals are based on a worldview in which the daily life of the community is affected by metaphysical agencies, in other words by gods, goddesses, and spirits. To enlist the aid of these agencies, or to mitigate their displeasure, shamans and other spiritual practitioners use a variety of technologies to gain access to what they conceive of as the "spirit world." There are rituals for fighting sorcery, locating "lost souls," for mobilizing community support for the indisposed, and for dozens of other desirable outcomes. Anthropologists have identified a typology of rituals, among them healing rituals (in which one's health is restored), calendrical rituals (in which seasons or other time spans are demarcated), commemorative rituals (ranging from paying homage to mythic events or remembering important anniversaries), initiatory rituals (in which someone gains entrance into the tradition of select group), transition rituals ("rites of passage" in which a child becomes an adult, or in which someone enters or leaves the world), ceremonial rituals (ceremonies in which a chief assumes power, a couple is joined in matrimony, or an exchange of goods is enacted), protective rituals (conducted for the purpose of warding off attacks from malevolent spirits, wild animals, an enemy tribe, etc.), celebratory rituals (honoring victory over a hostile group, success of a hunting expedition, winning an award or prize, or enjoying a simple or elaborate feast), and rituals of affliction (during which forgiveness or relief is begged from powerful "otherworldly" forces thought to have wreaked havoc on a clan or community).

Obviously, there are overlaps among these categories. Some writers would expand (or contract) this list, and others would make sharper distinctions between "rituals," "rites," and "ceremonies." Nonetheless, most of these rituals involve symbols (an image that is imbued with deeper meaning) and metaphors (activities imbued with deeper meaning). During a celebratory ritual, a laurel wreath (or a gold medal) might be given to a champion athlete. During a wedding ceremony, blankets (or rings) might be exchanged. During a transition ritual, the deceased might be placed on an elevated platform to be consumed by birds of prey (or placed in an underground vault as protection against rejoining Nature). A commemorative ritual might recall the "Passover" that spared the first-born Jews from Pharaoh's wrath (or wildly celebrate the advent of Lent duing Carnival or Mardi Gras).

This marvelous book provides its fortunate readers with first-person examples of many types of rituals, with an emphasis on those that lead to transformation and healing. Readers will be surprised to learn that rituals are not fossilized relics of an ancient past, but are enacted wittingly or unwittingly during the 21st century. They will also learn how to ritualize their lives, filling each day with more intention, lucidity, mindfulness, awareness, and joy. Eating a home-cooked meal can be a ritual. Watching a sunrise or sunset can be a ritual. Rituals are involved in sports events, in musical concerts, in scientific experiments, in sexual interactions, in worship services, and in visits to a physician's clinic or a psychotherapist's office. But gang wars, terrorist strikes, spousal abuse, and suicidal acts can be highly ritualized as well. Ritualization is morally and ethically neutral; it is up to the performer of the ritual to make it life-affirming or life-denying.

But life is filled with surprises. A young person on her way to medical school might attend a theatrical performance so moving that she switches college majors and becomes an actress. A successful warrior in Kenya might receive a "call" from the spirit world, give away his weapons, and apprentice himself to a shaman. A family determined to preserve its ethnic heritage may be shocked when a child elopes with a partner from another ethnicity, soon bringing home a beautiful golden-skinned baby who looks like nobody else in the family. But being mindful, by taking nothing for granted, and by paying attention to clues from society and from Nature, people can cope with a chaotic, unpredictable world and yet bring order out of chaos by constantly reframing, revising, and reinventing their lives.

Rituals are essential in this type of coping, whether one casts the coins of the I Ching, reads a spread of Tarot cards, or tosses the Rune stones or the Zulu bones. The ambiguous results of the resulting configurations allow unconscious solutions to perplexing problems to emerge, demonstrating that intentionality takes place not only at a surface level, but at more subtle and complex levels of the psyche. These rituals are not so much a matter or superstition or "magical thinking" as they are a way of allowing hidden patterns (what some people call "synchronicities") to come to emerge and expand possibilities and potential choices. Readers of this book may be told that these stories argue for "predestination," "fixed karma," or the negation of "free will." Don't believe them. The stories that Dr. Don Eulert and his crew have pulled together will help those who have lost their way to recover it, will assist those who feel a vacuum in their souls to discover fulfillment, and will provide inspiration to readers who have despaired when contemplating how their puny efforts can change their lives, much less their societies. This book and these stories can nourish the body, the mind, the spirit, or all three.

Sometimes I am called upon to throw coins for friends who want help from the I Ching in making a decision. Several years ago, a distraught college student asked me to obtain a hexagram from the I Ching to help her decide whether or not to continue her struggles with institutionalized education. For me, the verse was very clear, indicating that she should continue taking her courses, difficult though they were. For her the advice was also clear, and she decided to withdraw from school and join an artists' colony. I said nothing about my own interpretation because her own thinking had been clarified and she made the correct decision, as later events indicated.

Quite often, I will open a workshop with a Zulu ritual I learned during my visit to South Africa. I begin by having participants breathe into a pouch containing the imitation bones I had been given. Then I toss the bones, and one of 16 possible configurations emerges. I ask group members to interpret the resulting symbol as if it were a dream. If "the glittering stones" pattern was evoked, it might refer to the gems of wisdom people hope to obtain during the workshop. If "the journey" is the traditional appellation given to the four bones, participants might say that it refers to their personal quest for greater knowledge. But sometimes something more than projection seems to be at work. On one occasion, "the sound of the hammer" appeared; later that day, a group of carpenters started repair work on a nearby building and we heard hammering on and off for the remainder of the weekend. One time, "the rising snake" was the result of my toss. During the afternoon break, most of our participants went to the nearby river to wade or to swim. A young boy joined them, and within minutes a small snake slithered up his arm. He stood by in wonder as the snake wound its way toward his head. His parents panicked, screaming "Kill the snake!" But our workshop participants attempted to calm them down saying that the harmless creature was part of the pattern that was the logo of our workshop. In the meantime, the snake slid down the boy's neck and disappeared into the water. A year later, at the same location, the bones evoked "the little tree." A workshop participant left the room, returning a few minutes later with a flower pot containing a sprouting twig that she had taken, with permission, from one of the trees in the area where the Buddha reportedly had attained Enlightenment some 2,500 years earlier. I could give other examples, but those will suffice to demonstrate the limitations of the Western cause-and-effect worldview and its linear concept of time.

In 2011 I attended one of the most remarkable rituals of my life. Chief Pat Alfred of the Namgris tribe had died. His tribe is part of the Kwakwawa'wakw Nation in Eastern Canada, and for several years his relatives had prepared an elaborate ritual known as a "potlatch." This ritual involves a series of "giveaways" in honor of a fallen leader or respected tribal member. But in 1885 the government of British Colombia, Canada, outlawed these observances, considering them to be "pagan" and "non-Canadian." Once some of the First Nation people became lawyers and community organizers, considerable effort was put forward to reinstating these practices, which included a variety of healing rituals as well. When the 1885 law was repealed, the morale of the tribal men and women was enhanced and they returned to their traditional ways with gusto.

For me, it was a moving experience to observe the dances and dramatizations, each of which paid tribute to the late, beloved chief. There were various enactments during which tribal members wore the elaborate masks and garments that have brought recognition to these unique art forms. The director of a series of rituals portraying the "gathering of the animals" gifted me with a hand painted drum depicting the spirits of the sea. Badly abused as a child by members of the clergy who ran the school he was forced to attend, he told me how his healing took place after studying and observing his tribe's rituals – the same rituals that had been banned in the 1880s because they were considered "pagan." I remarked, "If this is paganism, let's have more of it!"

For those prospective readers who might reject a book about rituals because they are outdated relics of an irrational past, I would give the same rejoinder. The venerable story behind the ritual might not be historically or scientifically accurate, but this is not the essence of a ritual. A ritual's soul lies in is symbols, its metaphors, its meanings, and its intentions. Rituals are both process-oriented and goal-oriented. Each of the stories in this book is a gem. And this jewel-encrusted mosaic will reveal that ritual is alive and vital in the 21st century. It is ritual that will save the environment. It is ritual that will bring peace to our tattered world. It is ritual that will provide balance to people rent by trauma, depression, and anxiety. And we deny or overlook ritualized living at our peril.

1

BRINGING RITUAL TO LIFE

How to Ritualize Life

MALIDOMA SOMÉ ▮

I AM CALLED MALIDOMA, HE WHO IS TO "BE FRIENDS WITH THE stranger/enemy." (The word "doma" is used to refer to both meanings. The idea is that a stranger can become an enemy, and so a stranger is sacred because it is the task of him who is not a stranger to turn the potential enemy in the stranger into a friend.) In my many years since the passing of Grandfather, I have suffered greatly and learned greatly in the pursuance of what I see as my calling. Today, I wonder whether my life in exile makes me more of a stranger/enemy than one who would or should be friend, or should it be the other way round? The quest constantly imposing itself upon me has been more a quest for a home in the hearts of people — a thing that I take as a yardstick by which to measure the level of my own comfort — than a desire to efface myself behind the commonality of mechanistic standardization. And the constant questions ghostly looming in my consciousness are what can I tell my brothers and sisters across the great sea? How relevant is a small village in the wilds of Western Africa to the hustle and bustle of Western society? The West is crowded with people who want healing — this much I have been able to notice. There are people who know that somewhere deep within is a living being in serious longing for a peaceful and serene life. These are people who are so dissatisfied with the existing system that they will embrace anything that promises to rescue them from a sense of entrapment. Without real ritual there is only illness. Such illness cannot be healed with pills or drugs or alcohol, or shopping at the mall, or being tranced out many hours a day in front of the TV screen.

I started out in this book with a concern: where does this trouble in modern people come from? Being modern or Western does not mean being devoid of trouble. I have come to suspect that in the absence of ritual, the soul runs out of its real nourishment, and all kinds of social problems then ensue. I do not want to pretend that I can provide a model for fixing the ills of Western society. My intentions are much more modest. They are the results of my observations and experiences as a person caught in this culture and alienated by it. From the echoes of my ancestors, I feel I can give some clue as to how to improve that which is in constant decay in this culture. The truth is, I am also trying to make myself feel good by doing that which my own elders commissioned me to do. If my elders have deplored the sweeping effect of modernity, they have also lived in admiration of how effective news from the Otherworld, the primitive world, can help others understand and appreciate themselves better.

I suggest that the road to correcting ills goes through the challenging path of ritual. I suggest that ritual not be simply copied from one civilization to another but simply inspired by some culture still in touch with it. The soul of any man or woman craves for this touchstone to the inner self that puts us back in touch with our primal selves. In Western culture, the closest thing to ritual I have seen is liturgical ceremony, always charged with boredom, and in any case incomplete in what it seeks to accomplish — an intimacy with the Divine. Ceremony is only a component of ritual. Ritual is not just an elegant procession or music that lifts the soul or words that ordain.

To ritualize life, we need to learn how to invoke the spirits or things spiritual into our ceremonies. This means being able to pray out loud, alone. Invocation suggests that we accept the fact that we ourselves don't know how to make things happen the way they should. And thus we seek strength from the spirits or Spirit by recognizing and embracing our weakness. This way, before getting started with any aspect of our lives — travel, a project, a meeting — we first bring the task at hand to the attention of the gods or God, our allies in the Otherworld. We openly admit to them what we are facing and how overwhelming it is. By ritually putting what we do in the hands of the gods, we make it possible for things to be done better because more than we are involved in its getting done. Also, willingness to surrender the credit of our accomplishments to Spirit puts us in greater alignment with the Universe.

From an aboriginal point of view, no one can accomplish anything who is not in alignment with the gods or with a God. Anything created without the blessings of the gods or God comes loaded with ills. It does not take much time to send a little invocation at the start and at the end of the day. This way everything in between is sanctified or sacred and safer because it has been thrown into the hands of the spirit world. A person's life is ritualized who accepts the fact that everything he or she does is the work of the hands of the Divine. Everyone can do this. Anyone can, before going out in the morning, send a little prayer to the ancestors on the hills or in the river. It takes a word or two, or at most a few sentences. It is private and effective.

Modern communities can benefit from a good sense of ritual if they begin by experimenting with it emotionally. I don't think it is possible to be fully into ritual while one is carrying a load of undelivered emotions. The way you know that your rituals are having a positive effect on you begins with the discovery of how much emotion is pushing you from the inside like a volcano. Those who are able to express their emotions have been, at some point in their lives, in alignment with their own spirits, saints, guides or guardians.

Modernism means unemotionalism, or that which owes emotion to the world. It also means loss of memory of that way of acting that encompasses both the body and the soul. To cleanse the modern world from its unresolved problems of the soul, there ought not to be a Memorial Day but a massive funeral day when everyone is expected to shed tears for the titanic loss wrecked by Progress on people's souls. I have seen and or participated in some aspects of funerals or burial rites on a minuscule scale in this culture. What I saw was how difficult it is for the modern man to shed tears at length, and how everything that is done to encourage tears degenerates into some kind of strange liturgical solemnity that smells of repression or unwilinness to actually do that which is needed for release of deep grief.

I was once part of a grief ritual for Vietnam veterans. I went there bracing myself to face a flood of weeping eyes. A lot of people were there, more than I could count. But instead of an occasion for grieving, it was a ceremony almost similar to that which happens at Arlington Cemetery on Memorial Day. People showed up thinking this was going to be a good idea. They did not come out of a desire, to mourn. The setting was beautiful, the lights blinding, the electronic sound system deafening. It felt as if there were an edge of sensationalism, or solemnity, but no communal grief. The candle procession that followed on the wet road leading to the wharf was beautiful and elevating, not mournful. I remember seeing a repressed tear here and there and wondering why people behave as if it is illegal to cry their guts out. The grief ritual for Vietnam vets was in its intent a noble initiative that fell short of being able to pull the vets back home.

This experience led me to wonder whether it was possible to propose giving a Dagara-style funeral. Michael Meade, one of today's leading voices in men's consciousness and awareness — teacher of wisdom, artisan of symbols, metaphors and myth in the stories of humans — has always been in favor of rituals. He encouraged such a ritual at a men's conference. Of course a lot of the details in Dagara funerals were dropped due to the impossibility of applying them. Since nobody was supposed to be dead at the conference, death was symbolized. It was an innovation that worked just the same. What happened was that we contented ourselves with dividing the participants into three groups: the containers, the mourners or grievers, and the singers. The zeal with which people involved themselves was baffling.

Led by a master drummer, the singers were in ritual preparation long before the actual beginning of the ritual. Over the course of several days, they prayed, rehearsed and prayed again. The grievers were in real grief long before they got the permission to let loose. For three afternoons we gathered, prayed to the waters, the tears of Mother Earth shed so we might live in her lap. We told each other stories of loss, pain and frustration. The sincerity of the tellers authorized the grief of the group. Meanwhile, the containers busied themselves like ants, and with unparalleled dedication erected one of the most startling edifices which was to serve as the shrine and the border between this world and the next. In fact it was not an expensive-looking shrine, just a creative artifact brought to existence by the dedicated wit of its builders. It looked like an arch, or a dome with half of its size being an opening delineating this world and the next. It was made with the elements of nature: dry wood, leaves, grass. There was at the door a little space where, later on, people brought bundles symbolizing their losses. A few feet from it was a line separating the tribe of men from the Otherworld. Twenty feet away, there was a space specifically designated as the village where the grief was supposed to be held. The space in between constituted the road of grief, the place of chaos and commotion. It was made clear that anyone charged with grief should pull away from the village and carry his grief to the threshold and throw it in there, then come back to the village. People had the option to rush to the shrine, walk there or dance their way to it. The speed was a function of the emotional intensity. They were to be assisted by others who were instructed to stop them gently as they reached the line, wait for them to drop their grief into the Otherworld, then return to the village together. Every expression of emotion was supposed to be done facing the shrine.

When the ritual actually began, there was genuineness everywhere. The genuineness quickly translated into an appalling chaos everywhere. First, there were more mourners than helpers. Loads of them packed themselves up at the shrine. Fascinated by the sight of the Otherworld, they were unwilling to return to the village. Worse, some of them, mesmerized by the beyond, wanted to throw themselves into it as if in serious need to join the dead.

Second, it was impossible to trust that the line of demarcation was going to be observed. The pull of the Otherworld was powerfully visible. The interdiction to cross the line was enforced by guards. They used their fists at times to bounce contorted grieving bodies back to the village. Some people who were asked to return to the village felt hurt. They thought it meant that once again it was not OK to grieve. So they turned around and mourned their way back to the village. I was appalled. Normally, from an indigenous point of view, if you want to know where a funeral shrine is, follow a griever. This time it did not work. How did it happened that the village was turned into a shrine?

The implications were so heavy I could barely believe my eyes. Michael and I ran everywhere, like men from the fire department battling a blaze. Someone had to explain in gentle terms to these sincere people the need to avoid throwing their grief at the living. Meanwhile, grievers, torn by a flood of unleashed grief and mortally attracted by the beyond, symbolized by the shrine, attacked the guards who were posted at the threshold to prevent them from jumping into the Great Beyond. They could not resist the pull from the beyond. Honest screaming souls leapt toward the shrine — they had become the bundle. They were recuperated by strong hands and sent back to the village side. As if feeling defied, they gathered their forces together and leapt back only to find themselves reminded in an equal way that they did not belong to the Otherworld yet, and that the village needed them. Other grievers were angry; they ejaculated some insanities at the shrine, screaming at the tops of their voices and ending with a torrential weeping that would break the heart of the toughest CEO. It was no longer a Dagara grief ritual, but a ritual — period. People leapt out of the village in single line and danced their way to the shrine, turned around and came back home to the village. It was beautiful to see. The space between the village and the shrine was busy. The cleansing was happening. So much grief surfaced that the shrine was jam-packed with a crowd of men who did not quite register that they were only supposed to go to the shrine and drop their grief and return to the village where the drumming and the chanting was going on. The containers' job had to be edited a little bit to clean it of its therapist-like influence. Besides these little cultural infiltrations, it was a small success. I saw hot tears flowing from wet eyes. That felt good. I heard sincere groans and yells and screams that almost made me feel like I was home again. The ritual was working.

Even though it was just scratching the surface, the scratch was at least opening something. In a way, there was an invitation to unleash grief. The experience left people empty, light, and — above all — miraculously prone to celebrate. I understood why, in the village, life rotates around grief and celebration. People celebrate because they have paid their dues to the dead. The other side of real grief is real joy. Unfinished grief trans-lates into petty joy and silly amusement. The experience taught me a great deal. Without ritual, humans live in nostalgia.

When there is an opportunity for people to mourn their losses, the horizon for rites that heal will be pure and bright, and healing will come pouring into the souls in a great moment of reunion.

Can I impart to the modern world that which is rooted in the ancestral world? Only time will tell. I offer the tales of Grandfather and Guisso to serve as a testament to what rests in the aboriginal soul. Are we not of a common soul as proposed by modern thinkers such as Jung? If so, then what serves the soul of the Dagara may well prove to resonate in the soul of modern peoples also. And so I offer the prayer to our common ances-tors on behalf of those seeking to recover themselves from the rubble of modernity as they seek to work their way toward being elders of the new post-modern tribal order.

May the spirits of every pertinent direction take notice of their hearts' desire.

May the forces below pump strength into their feet — that they walk the walk of their life, the walk that heals the wounded truth of their bellies and keeps the eyes of their memory open so they can grow niyang maru.

May the ancestral fuel burn in their spiritual veins and animate their souls with vision so they can hold hands niyang maru.

As they walk toward their future,

May they wake up fast to the dialogue between the soul and the spirit.

And may they labor to clean the world from its paralyzing epidemic of soul-barrenness so that tomorrow our children can sing together in peace.

THE PRAYER OF FAITH

GAIL REINER

THE TRAILBLAZER OF FAITH AND DAILY PRAYER IN OUR FAMILY WAS MY great-grandmother Ida Olson. As a child growing up in Finland she learned to read from the Bible, a primer in the small rural school she attended through the completion of her education in 4th grade. One day, when she was around eight years old, after reading the ten commandments in Exodus 20 she went to the calendar and said to her mother, "Mama, we are worshipping on the wrong day", to which her mother replied, "shush."

After immigrating to America as a young woman she welcomed a door-to-door Bible salesman into her home one day. After praying together and talking, she learned that he was a Seventh-Day Adventist (SDA). As he shared the SDA doctrines of worshipping on Saturday as the Sabbath of creation, in honor of the fourth commandment and the day that Jesus worshipped, she realized this was the religion she had been seeking since early childhood. Soon after she was baptized into the SDA faith.

Although I never met her, I loved to hear my mother tell stories about how people would come for miles to have her pray with them because her prayers were so heart-felt and beautiful. At seventy-four, as Grandma Olson lay dying in the hospital, one of the attending physicians quietly lifted the sheets on her bed to show the young residents the calluses on her knees from the hours she spent kneeling in prayer.

For me, growing up in a very imperfect but loving Seventh-Day Adventist (SDA) home, prayer and Bible reading were a vital part of everyday life. Big "AMENS" came from the congregation in church on Sabbath morning after I recited with my girlish voice a string of memory verses from the Bible. In my early years, the memory verses might be short for easy and successful recall such as the first portion of Daniel 6:22: "My God hath sent his angel, and hath shut the lions' mouths..." which provided a strong visual reminder of the power of angels to save life if directed by God.

I attended church school where we were required to memorize entire passages such as the original King James Bible version of the Ten Commandments. In one church college religion class, the course grade was contracted according to the number of Bible texts each student committed to memory. Other church rituals such as baptism by immersion (when we were old enough to understand and to request it) and foot washing before communion service, only became peculiar to me when I realized that not all the neighborhood children did these things in their churches or synagogues.

During a period when we were each going through divorce, an old high school friend David and I re-connected in 1999 after not having seen each other for decades. Mutual consolation turned our renewed friendship to romantic love and we married in the outdoor wedding of my dreams at the Navy Seal base in Coronado in 2002. In our adult years both Dave and I had fallen or run away from the faith of our youth. We made a million excuses why church didn't make sense to us: social shunning from our churches during divorce, living lifestyles contrary to how we'd been raised, poor preaching and unfriendly congregations were a few of the complaints we shared. Secretly we each felt a persistent loneliness for God. We desired a forum for worshipping with other like-minded believers who really had embraced the beliefs of our religion.

My return to God began when I was working per diem as a bedside nurse. One patient I had was a Filipina Catholic woman in her late 50s. She was dying of colon cancer and was declining rapidly with only days to live. During one particular day I cared for her, family who had flown into San Diego from all over the world to pay their respects to their beloved auntie crowded into her room. I had never seen so many family members come to see any patient before. Late afternoon as she began to tire they left to make their way to their hotels. I sat on her bed and asked her what it had been like to be at the receiving end of so much respect and love. She was eager to talk, and her eyes filled with tears as she told me how she had been the auntie in the family who had never married in order to care for elderly parents. After her parents both died, she lovingly cared for nieces and nephews who stayed with her in Manila while they studied at University. She said that she had been glad for the life that she had lived and felt proud of everything she had contributed to the family, and that she was not crying from loss but from regret.

She asked if I remembered one young woman who had sat in the corner of her room who had been exceptionally quiet. I remembered her distinctly, a pretty young woman in her early 20s with a sweet smile. As I described her correctly, my patient shared that she had never accepted this niece or treated her as nicely as she had her other nieces and nephews because this niece had been adopted and was not related "by blood." I felt honored that she would share the guilt and sadness she felt over this mistake, which was so deeply painful. Clearly this niece had coped, moving forward in achieving her goals--she was a medical student in New York, but still my patient was grieving her own hardness of heart. As her tears turned into stifled sobs, without even realizing why, out of my mouth came a memory verse from college, John 14:1-3 "Let not your heart be troubled: ye believe in God, believe also in me. In my Father's house are many mansions: if it were not so, I would have told you. I go to prepare a place for you. And if I go and prepare a place for you, I will come again, and receive you unto myself; that where I am, there ye may be also." As I finished sharing this promise she clutched my hand in astonishment and shouted "the Lord Jesus Christ sent you here Himself today!" I hugged her and held her for a few moments, sharing a feeling of peaceful closeness. Before long I excused myself fled to the bathroom, shaking with an almost paralyzing shame. Like the apostle Peter before the crucifixion, I had denied my Lord, yet Jesus had not denied me, He had continued to use me to bring love and comfort to the dying. My patient died peacefully two days later surrounded by family.

A few months later, my mother came for a visit during the winter holiday season to escape rainy dark Seattle. It was her practice to go to church every Sabbath. We decided we would attend church with her. The church closest to our home is South Bay SDA church. It's a very small church that is multicultural without trying, a kaleidoscope of Hispanics, Blacks, Asians, Filipinos and a handful of Whites. Despite the small size of the congregation, they lifted the rafters during hymn singing. A member of the youth group , gave the sermon. She spoke on the closeness you can have with God when you bring your troubles to Him even during your darkest times. We were amazed to see the deep belief, not only of this young woman, but also of all the youth who, unlike youth of many churches who sit on the last rows of the sanctuary, sat on the front pews, Bibles open. We were instantly hooked; it was the church home that we had been secretly longing for.

A week later we had the privilege of hearing Pastor James Robins preach. Having tragically lost an infant daughter during a car crash in which he and the baby's mother were also injured, and after years of encouraging his son who had a life-changing stroke, he was no stranger to suffering. After his sermon on God's faithfulness, and unknown to my husband, I slipped into his office to share my desire for rebaptism.

Two weeks later Pastor Robins preached again, this time on putting God to the test. Dave grew pale and quiet during the call at the end of the message as he stood up to indicate his willingness to put God to the test. No one in that audience but I knew that the test he was putting God to was to take away the craving and habit of marijuana use that had held him captive for 30 years. No one would have guessed, as he was on the medical faculty of a major university, a research scientist in infectious disease biology. Dave got his miracle, and both the craving and the habit left that day. In March 2003 we entered the baptismal together to affirm our commitment to live out our lives as Seventh Day Adventist Christians.

In 2004, just over a year after our baptism, we were on vacation in New Hampshire. I woke up early in the morning urgently requesting to go to the E.R. of the closest hospital we could find. Unexplained fatigue, and ultimately excruciatingly painful bladder and rectal spasms and urinary

urgency, had been misdiagnosed for over a year as urinary tract infec-
tions. I began to think that I was psychosomatically sympathizing with
a beloved ovarian cancer patient. The E.R. physician was thorough, and
looked very serious when he came to talk about my abdominal CAT scan
results. He indicated that I had cysts on my ovaries large enough to recommend surgery as soon as possible. He gave us the option of staying
there for surgery or, with the help of pain medication, returning to California for surgical care closer to home. I elected for the latter option,
reassured that they were just "large cysts"-- not realizing until later reflection that when I had said, "man, I thought I had ovarian cancer" that the
physician had looked away.

When I got back to California my primary care doctor was unable to
open the CD of my CAT scan on her computer, so I called the radiology
department of the New Hampshire hospital to request they fax the ra-
diologist's interpretation to my office. They were very accommodating
and faxed the report immediately. I stood in shock at the fax machine at
work as I read the interpretation summary for myself: "ovarian cancer."
I'd seen patients die of ovarian cancer, including my own grandmother,
and it can be a very difficult downward slope towards death. I was scared.

As Dave and I selectively shared the shocking news of my cancer with
family and a few friends, one friend, gospel singer Veronica Abell, immediately suggested that I have an anointing service. Based on the Biblical
teaching in James 5:14, 15 "Is any sick among you? let him call for the
elders of the church; and let them pray over him, anointing him with oil
in the name of the Lord; And the prayer of faith shall save the sick, and
the Lord shall raise him up; and if he have committed sins, they shall be
forgiven him." The anointing service is not reserved for the dying, but is
performed for anyone seriously ill who requests it.

A week after the anointing service I had surgery. Dr. Ed Bryan, a chap-
lain and psychologist who had done pre-marriage counseling for us, came
to the hospital to pray with us. Dave and I touched on our understanding
that healing can come in many forms. Having both been academics for
over 20 years, my husband and I had done a lot of reading on ovarian cancer, and we understood that tumors over 10 cm were often associated with

poor outcomes. We were also concerned that my Ca-125, a blood marker for cancer, was nearly 500 when normal is below 35. The surgeon came out of the operating room to tell Dave and the family that he discovered I had two tumors that had linked in the center, with its overall size about 15 cm. He was pleased to report that it appeared not to have spread.

Some people wonder why, if God healed, I still had a tumor. They wonder why I underwent five treatments of chemotherapy, three of which had to be done in hospital because I suffered such severe side effects. I believe that whatever we have to endure in this life, it is all for the glory of God. And as long as I had strength to smile and encourage others, I kept on trying. During the weeks and months I had on the couch, learning how to be rather than do, I listened to the Bible on CD. My "chemo" memory verse was Psalms 46:10 "Be still, and know that I am God." I rested in the knowledge that I was loved and that this is not the only life we get. I shifted from having meaning and purpose in my life, too dependent on contributing to the lives of family, friends and even myself, toward gaining a sense of purpose from reflection, meditation and prayer; feeling the sun on my face, noticing the depth of color in a flower, the patterns of leaves on the tree outside my study window and the treasured concern of paw checks from my Labradors.

This shift from doing to being is perhaps one of the most difficult challenges any person who has endured cancer, or any other debilitating illness, is faced with. Hope shifts during these experiences from hoping to contribute to hoping that we will navigate the course of our illness with grace and flexibility and yes, even honesty, about how we feel.

Throughout my illness my husband was attentive and caring, always willing to be present, sharing what wisdom he felt he could offer. When my once shoulder-length hair was cropped short and then began to fall like rain on my pillow, it was time to get the razor out. Dave determined we needed the #1 setting, the setting he'd once used when son Alex was in football. Losing my hair was one of the easiest things for me, and we laughed through the entire process.

The good-humored coping and positive attitude I showed during initial phase of my illness was not easily sustained during progressive hospitalizations and worsening side effects from chemotherapy. One night my energy was so low I didn't know it was possible to be that tired. I felt that I was dying. Dave, whose usual answer for most illnesses is to take a hot bath and sleep, prescribed these two measures for me. Being just days away from my final chemotherapy, however, I told him that I wanted to just try and enjoy myself for a little bit while I still could. He looked at me over his glasses, got up from his chair, and without saying a word put music on and pulled me up to dance with him closely and wordlessly for an hour and a half.

That evening I went from hoping that time would move past my final chemo at the speed of light, to wishing it would stand still forever in that slow dance. I learned, in those moments of receiving, the power of a loving word, a kind look, and focused attention. I hoped that somehow in our closeness Dave could feel my gratitude. I often hope that the attitude of gratitude for life I've developed as a benefit from having suffered is something I will never forget.

When circumstances cause us to do a life review and to think about what our life has been all about, the hope to leave a legacy becomes an internal ritual of sorts. The dictionary defines a legacy as "something handed down from an ancestor or predecessor from the past." It gives "a legacy of religious freedom" as an example. As we become acutely aware of our mortality and whether or not we hope for a future in heaven, most of us hope to leave something behind that marks in some way that we were loving and helpful, that we made a positive impact while we were here. I thank God now that our children have the greatest legacy we could hope for, a spirit of love and the courage to serve others.

For me the rituals of Bible study and memorization, prayer, baptism, communion, Sabbath-keeping and anointing are beautiful symbols of a relationship with a loving God who loves me now and who will love me forever when, as He promised in John 14, He will come again. I have been deeply touched, since my cancer diagnosis, by friends and family from many faiths and philosophies performing rituals of their own to signify their love. One Catholic brother-in-law, Al, and other Catholic friends have often lit candles at mass on my behalf, Sri Lankan Buddhist friends pray for me and shocked us during my time in chemotherapy with an amazing financial gift to cover co-pays for medications. I have a photo of one best friend, an atheist, cleaning my kitchen in her bikini. Another best friend and her mother made a beautiful sea-theme quilt which comforted me during every hospitalization and continues to warm me each night. Sisters bathed me, changed my sheets, cooked; brothers sent food. My mother would burst into prayer when we talked on the phone.

I am profoundly blessed to be so loved and supported. It is my daily prayer that I will continue to celebrate loving relationships each day in this life, showing love even to those who aren't always so nice. I look forward to the life to come where there will be no more pain, sadness, sickness or death. Even so come, Lord Jesus.

WITH RITUALS LARGE AND SMALL WE HEAL, WE RE-MEMBER

FRANCESCA CIANCIMINO HOWELL

RITUAL IS AN ESSENTIAL PART OF HUMAN LIFE, JUST AS IT IS PART OF nonhuman or the more-than-human life. Our most ancient brains not only understand but also seem to crave ritual. Weaving ritual into our lives gives life a wholeness, a completeness, mending the ragged ends back together. Ritual returns to us a shape that life has lost, a meaningfulness we knew in our hearts had to be there.

As one who has spoken various languages throughout life, with professional careers on three continents, and for whom English is an art as well as a means of communication, I love to play with words and examine their meanings. So, if I play with the word remember and say that rituals help us "re-member", it helps to express the feeling that rituals bring back integral parts of ourselves-- reconnecting us, renewing bonds. Performing a familiar ritual, a time-honored one, not only makes the mundane sacred once more, but also makes us feel safe, in a strange inexplicable way.

I am truly a person of rituals, both large and small. Of course, one could say that no ritual is small – because each and every one brings soothing or meaning or answers a need. However, when I say I am a person of ritual, I also mean it more formally: I am a Priestess of the earth-based pagan religion known as Wicca. In American Judeo-Christian society, I have sometimes described myself as a "pre-Christian Minister" to impart the seriousness of the commitment and sense of service. My life has held myriad rituals, whether joining in as participant or as officiator for weddings, dedications, baby blessings, memorials and many others.

Thus, I have spent a large part of recent years creating rituals for my community, in groups both large and small, spending hours reading over other people's rituals, and days and nights helping them to create them. Given that I am also a wife and mother, I have spent my adult life creating rituals in the family to bring special meaning and beauty to the changing phases of the seasons, to shared meals, to our home and-- quite simply put-- to life.

There it is, in its barest essence. Rituals heal by bringing meaning back to life. Even animals incorporate ritual into their lives, consciously or unconsciously. Ritual actions weave meaning and comfort into our lives in ways that we may not even be conscious of. Does an atavistic sense call us to repeat things that worked before for survival reasons? Perhaps. Whatever the reason, there is a sense of keen satisfaction when a ritual goes well – when accomplished with a group, it is as though a sense of joy is shared in the "tribe." These are powerful emotions, touching life into a truly pre-modern part of one's soul, as ritual must. We postmodern people crave these connections and re-memberings – events and moments that give us back the bits of our souls we have allowed to be fragmented by the pace and brutality of postmodern life. The honoring of ritual with a group also creates or re-affirms the bonds of community, an act which is healing in itself. Rituals heal by bringing us back to our deeper selves, responding to our most ancient nature, to a need for wellbeing in a bare-bones, tribal, pre-modern sense. Ritualizing our lives answers some of humanity's earliest needs. In this way they make us feel safe: we believe that life will go on if I do this.

I lived in Colorado for thirteen years, where I led two covens, taught classes on many topics, including Wicca, and was involved integrally in the Unitarian-Universalist Church. There I had a role in helping the ministers and congregations to create ceremonies of many kinds. Although I currently live in Italy, I keep in close touch with my community there and keep my "practice" of Wicca going here.

While living in Colorado I was consistently impressed by the powerful hunger in people at certain times of the year, and in certain times of their lives, pointing to unanswered longing for ritual in postmodern human souls. The Winter Solstice is one of the clearest examples. It is a time when people's hearts long for quiet and beauty, away from the consumer frenzy that nowadays accompanies Christmas, Hanukah and other seasonal commemorations in December. Men and women alike, old and young, love the sense of the numinous, of the magic that can come with observing the longest night of the year. (They also love the joy that can come in observing the shortest night of the year -- Summer Solstice is another ancient festival that I found people resonate to and revel in.) In my experience people were absolutely delighted to be invited to participate in a Winter Solstice ritual, whether it was small enough to fit in my living room, or whether it was a large ceremony.

A friend of mine, a dancer and movement therapist in Colorado, began her own annual Winter Solstice gatherings at about the same time I began my rituals. Hers were more informal than mine, but no less magical. She would gather a few like-minded friends who brought musical instruments, a piece of poetry or writing, and some food and wine or other drinks to share. In a beautifully decorated home, amidst candlelight and seasonal symbols, people would sit on the floor, read or say some poetry or pieces pertinent to the night of the Solstice, ("Yule" in the northern European traditions), and sing some songs as well. Music of some form usually plays an important part. There is a power in singing together, when people "drop" into a shared sense of being present fully to a moment in time. Breathing together, letting go of mundane thoughts, stress and worrying, for precious minutes, THIS is the power and beauty of ritual: creating time outside of time, a time that is no time. Those concepts are part of Wicca, where we insist that no watches or clocks be present in a Wiccan ritual, to symbolize that fully.

The Yule or Winter Solstice rituals I created and led offered a more formal version. We would write the ceremony carefully, and those participating learned their lines. We often enacted something known in psychology as a "psycho-drama": a symbolic, traditional representation of a legend or well-known fable. Sometimes we used a common legend much performed in Wicca, of a battle between a young king and an old king. In essence the Waning Year that battles the new Waxing Year for power and authority in the months to come. At Winter Solstice the Young Lord who wins is the "Oak King", and thus the Wheel of the Year turns, and Spring will once more win out over Winter in the months to come. (It is the opposite at Summer Solstice).

Another year, being a bit tired of the usual battle enactment, I researched a legend that had piqued my curiosity and called to me: the Lord of Misrule. A mischievous jester then graced our Circle that year, with riddles and jests for those who attended – evoking a traditional European custom of the winter holidays whose roots go back many centuries.

Such stories and legends have universal archetypal meanings, another factor that resonates deep in our primitive, unconscious minds. As we gather to celebrate the turning of the wheel of the year, speaking words together and singing songs rich in symbolism and in archetype, a healing power washes over the participants. Rituals of this nature give back a profound quality to the seasons' changes, some of which, like the winter holidays or Halloween (another lovely ancient celebration) have been degraded by frenetic activity and unleashed consumerism. We buy, race, compete . . . futilely attempting to create the "perfect moment."

Rather than a better toy, elaborate decorations or glamorous gifts, what our souls and hungry hearts crave is a shared ritual experience with deep, complex symbols. We seek a simple and powerful moment that allows us to participate in the fear and awe that the darkest night of the year must have meant for our ancestors. What awe and ineffable relief must have flooded through the tribe and community when the Sun came up again! Did our ritual, our watching through the night bring the Sun back? Did our long past ancestors believe that? Maybe. Whatever the case, we felt safe once more. "Safe" in our shared act of gathering together, of calling out to the celestial, more-than-human beings, safe due to our careful observing of the holy night and holy event.

Ceremony and ritual evoke images that are lit by candles indeed have a powerful effect on a moment. The simple act of lighting a candle brings a holiness – wholeness – and a re-membering to an otherwise mundane or everyday event. Our family has often remarked on my consistent lighting of candles at dinner, and how it marks and even heightens the importance of our sitting down to share a meal together. Ancient symbolism and ancient chords are struck, which may well be the echo of our ancestors' sharing fire. We sit around our tables with candlelight as we once sat sharing life-giving fire. And thus the survival-driven act of eating is marked as holy . . . which indeed it is, as we share our food, share of our days, share our thoughts.

In my family the evening ritual is almost an unbreakable custom: we light candles and say grace, in a simple but meaningful way every night. Not only on significant dates or big holidays, not just when the extended family is present, but every night. No TV, no answering the phone, no loud music. Quiet, talking together, candles and grace. I believe that this small but extraordinarily powerful ritual has in itself contributed far-reaching healing on our little nuclear family. We are safe. We hold each other and honor each others' days, contributions, needs. As we join hands, we re-member after the day's travels. We send our thoughts to those we love or those in need, near and far. We perform an ancient daily ritual and it heals us.

Living in Italy now I see that this is a normal part of Italian life. I see this enduring custom in Italian society as contributing to emotional and psychological health here, often missing in America. Americans are not so apt to sit down and eat together on a regular basis as in other cultures, and that simple ritual would aid the country in significant ways.

Children and animals understand ritual. I have observed them creating rituals large and small, and relishing the observance of them. As a young person I attended Catholic Mass with my family, a meaningful community ritual which my mother never missed. In Catholicism there are many annual and seasonal observances that impacted my psyche in sweet, memorable ways, and which no doubt have had an impact on my creation of rituals as an adult. And as a young girl, on the more "mun-

dane" everyday level, I also cared for my horse all the years I was growing up, with the daily ritual of brushing him and carefully saddling him
before riding. He knew the daily routine with me. When it was time to
clean his hooves, he would lift them for me to pick out the debris. When
we were all finished and he was ready to go back to the field or barn, he
waited for the treats he knew were to come. (And which no doubt he felt
he deserved!)

My own children would build little "altars" in the woods or yard with
sticks and shells, rocks and flowers, as they commemorated or memorial-
ized some event or special intention. On some level they also understand
the healing, intrinsic nature of bringing ritual into daily life. In our family we always buried our deceased animal companions with proper fune-
real solemnity. Even the dead birds or mice which we sometimes found
in the garden received similar attentions. There is no doubt in my mind
that the performance not only eased the children's grief at the loss of our
non-human family member (and my own grief too), but also mended
the greater fabric of life and energy a bit, as each life was honored and
returned with ceremony to Mother Gaia.

I remember the old horse that always walked the same path down to
his favorite grazing spot each morning. I watch my cats stretch and stroll
to the same exact spot on the deck or the rug each day. In the same the
way I start my mornings with little personal rituals: greet the morning
and the family, walk to the kitchen for tea, pick up the paper, etc., etc.
Same actions, same sense of reassuring ourselves that "all's right with the
world." Is it our ancient reptilian brain that conditions us to perform
these repeated actions formally in ritual? If so, then perhaps rituals connect to a sense of survival and safety where repetition is necessary to ensure life's perpetuation. We reunite the pieces of our lives and traditions
with the repeated actions. These elements of ritual make us happy and
whole... heal us.

The healing elements of ritual large and small-- alone, at home, or
in the greater community-- come through repetition, but most importantly through mindfulness and awareness. They are not routines in a
rote, mindless sense. In ritual, those involved are made to feel safe, loved,

heard and held – whether human child, human adult or non-human family. Helping, healing, making life kinder and more complete – that is what caring means. In the formal sense of ritual and ceremony, I have witnessed the healing that comes through gentle touch and attention as we hold hands in community, we listen, we honor each other, we pause to see the sacred in the mundane. Through rituals large and small, simple and elaborate, we weave together once more the pieces of life, bringing the circle back together to wholeness, to healing, and to re-membering.

The Best Ritual of Them All: Mealtimes

Gary W. and Ann W. Lawson

When I was young and living at home, I never thought of meal times as a ritual. In fact, I thought very little about meal times, other than perhaps I had better be there on time. There were only two legs on that chicken and there were four kids who all liked chicken legs. If you were late you might end up with the back or the wings. I didn't need to think about meal time because meal times were predictable, always there, always on time. Dinner at 6:00 p.m., breakfast at 7:00 a.m. If it is Wednesday, we are more likely than not to have meatloaf. Sunday after church was pot roast, Monday was tuna casserole, and so on. My mom wasn't the kind to experiment with new recipes. In fact, in Tulsa in the late 50's when the first pizza place opened, I asked if we could go and was told, "You wouldn't like it. It's too spicy."

Much later in life, to my surprise, I found out my mom didn't even like to cook. Mealtime was something to get through, because it was expected. I now know the importance of those meals. I know how important they were for my family and especially to my father. Not that he ever talked about that. He was more of an action guy, not a talking guy (which wasn't unusual for men back then or even now). He never talked about his childhood, with the exception of the story about coming from Arkansas to Oklahoma in a covered wagon. It was hard for me to believe that then, though I know it was true.

I think the reason he didn't talk about his childhood was that it was not too pleasant, and the last thing he wanted to do was rehash it. His mom was often ill and died early, while he was in high school. There were eight children and an alcoholic father. According to stories from my aunts and uncles, life was often chaotic. Not the kind of environment you would wish for as a kid. So my dad did exactly what many people do-- create for your children the childhood you wished for as a child. His main issues in life were stability and predictability. (Perhaps that explains why I moved seventeen times, and lived in seven states and five European countries the first eighteen years I was married). I craved excitement and unpredictability. We often want what we don't have.

The one thing we did not do much of, as I was growing up, was to eat out. I remember the first McDonalds in Tulsa. After it opened I would pass it each day as I went to school. I wanted to eat there all the time. We as a family ate there one or two times a year. After I got my paper route and had some money of my own, I often ate there. I don't think my parents knew how much of my meager income I spent on junk food. It was my money and they let me spend it as I pleased for the most part.

My mom did get very upset the summer after my senior year in high school when I spent most of the money I had saved for college on a guitar. It as a slightly used Fender Stratocaster and it cost me the grand sum of $185. That was a lot of money then. A hamburger cost 15 cents. That guitar would be worth thousands now. And it turned out that I made thousands of dollars with that guitar to help pay for my college education. But, that's another story.

After I married my high school sweetheart in 1967, and we established our own home, we continued my family's tradition of regular mealtimes, especially dinners. I did not know at that time, or perhaps I knew at some level, that having dinner as a family was as important to my new bride as it had been for my father.

You see, my wife lived in a situation not unlike my father, where not much was predictable except unpredictability. There were many times after my wife's parents were divorced that she and her younger brother were left to fend for themselves at mealtime. Being the resourceful fifth grader that she was, she would take some money from her mothers purse, and she and her brother would walk to the local Dairy Queen for a fast food dinner.

So there is the dynamic in a nutshell. I longed for some excitement and had all of the predictability I could stand. She longed for some predictability and had more excitement than she could stand. It worked this way. She was attracted to me (my family) because of the stability, yet she was able to put up with and sometimes even enjoy my unpredictable side. I truly needed someone who would put up with me but would set some limits, yet someone who appreciated the exciting side of me. She was that person.

The ritual that pulled the entire thing together was dinner as a family. Whether it was as a couple when we were first married or later with our two kids, she insisted we sit down at mealtime. Not just to eat, but to talk and enjoy each other. Find out what was going on with each other, you know, keep in touch. I of course insisted we eat out once in a while, and I did not mind in the least her liberal use of spices. Turns out I did like pizza.

So what was it like having the Dr's Lawson for parents? According to our reasonably adjusted adult children, it was not too bad. They report feeling that they had the best of both worlds: regular meal times and a bit of excitement now and then. We almost always took them out with us when we went out to dinner, in some cases to very nice restaurants. The rule was, Behave or be taken to the car where you stay alone for the remainder of dinner. I only had to do that once with my son and twice with my daughter. They know how to behave, and they know how to get safely wild and have a good time once in awhile.

It makes me sad to think about all of the children who do not get a chance to experience the family mealtime ritual. I am afraid that we pay a price for having pizza delivered and eating it in front of the television, watching American Idol. Not speaking to each to hear How was your day? Too many busy parents don't even eat with their kids. (Perhaps that explains the popularity of the Food TV channel with all those cooking shows).

So here was and is our evening ritual. First, turn off the TV. Someone sets the table while everyone helps in some way to prepare the meal. Preferably eat at the dining room table, and use the good silverware. That's what it's there for. Have some wine, if you so choose. Children may have a taste if they like, and most often they don't like it. It won't be a big deal when they become teenagers, and some peer says "Let's sneak out and drink some alcohol". They can say "Been there done that. Don't need to sneak, no big deal." Add some mood music if you like, and don't forget the candles. They make every meal special.

Grab a fork. enjoy the meal . . . and talk! If you do that you have yourself a daily ritual that is not only enjoyable but healthy, both physically and psychologically. If you can't do it every day, do it more days than not. Now that the kids are grown and married, we have a dance or two to add to our already special ritual.

This ritual works not only for us. Research studies have demonstrated myriad benefits. Rituals such as dinnertime create resilience in children of alcoholics (with families who maintained their rituals in the face of active alcoholism in the family much less likely to transmit alcoholism to their children). The New York Times reported that frequent family meals were associated with a lower risk of children smoking, drinking and using marijuana. These children also had less depressive symptoms and suicidal thoughts, and much better grades. Another study found that, among families who had two or fewer dinners a week, teenagers were more than one and a half times as likely to smoke, drink and use drugs, compared to families who had five to seven dinners a week. Teens who had more family dinners were less likely to have sexually active friends, less likely for girls to have boyfriends two or more years older, and less time spent with boyfriends or girlfriends. Another study found that adolescent girls who had frequent family meals (that created a pleasant atmosphere) were less likely to have eating disorders.

So, enjoy your family dinner rituals! (And, and prevent problems common in our current culture).

The Sunset Becomes A Burning Temple, Pulses Light

Don Eulert

--Leave-taking poem for Larry Shaefer

When the sun is set, and the moon is set, and the fire has gone out,
and speech is hushed, what then is the light of man? <u>Upanishads</u>

Come ceremonial need-fire/wood
ritual, matter has grown cold; my
father's yearly festival with earth is lost

We would
put our hands on old rhythms, move
        toward another season

Put the firestick now to the forehead
draw the smoke into the mind
blow it to earth, to wind,
to midnight water;

In the night I tremble, knees and elbows
and forehead on the floor;
There is no single wisdom

Your stomach heaves
    as if it could empty you of pain;
you suffer defeat/ she cries out from darkness
we offer sacrifice   it belongs to
    no particular thing   it all comes in:
we can die without purpose
we answer love with selfishness, I
    don't know how to help you
"we are weak and poor,
we don't know anything"

Ourselves charged, how else should you learn
fire-boring , rhythmic motions
   spiritual feeding from breasts, the
woman sobbing from the candled dark

We discover ritual   it gives form
    to our suffering   it remembers
    what we are, who would forget:
our humility shapes to a waiting bowl

Then as it happens   just before dawn
she brings into this house earth
you bring the bowl for fire

We speak of suffering
we thus make fire with our mouths

Everyday Attentions to the Sacred

Paula Rosas

Every Monday all 1,200 of us silently sang. We wore our gala uniforms, were perfectly groomed, and smelled fresh with body lotion, shampoo, and gel. The sweet, sweet voice of Mother Lupita gently started the singing, and we all followed.

Mondays were the day of the Holy Spirit, and we invoked it with plenty of love. Perfect not to have my heavy backpack, have my body free, and just stand there in rows with all of my friends and schoolmates, singing. I suppose the song could be heard because we were many children, but I can't remember hearing it. We all sang immersed, but in some way I remember that it was completely silent. The world just stopped. I felt an immense peace, and everything felt in order and utterly safe. This ritual was religious, but it went beyond religion, beyond beliefs. It was really sacred. The school building remained the same, the voices were still present, we were all in our places, but we were all connected "through", "by" something more powerful, nonmaterial, something "greater", something "outside." But at the same time we were extremely present "inside" and could feel the fresh morning air traveling through our noses and bodies. Every Monday morning, during nine childhood years, many others and I felt this way.

I know there are many definitions of what is a ritual. Some scholars argue that the word should be rite; others view a ritual as a ceremony, while others insist they are different terms and should not be confused. I am not sure where that stands, but I do have my ideas as to what a ritual is. In my life, ritual is an experience that we perform on purpose to connect us to the spiritual realm, to our ultimate reality.

I believe rituals are an expression of our spiritual human quality. They are part of our desire to transcend and to feel that there is more to our existence than our individual self. Certainly rituals have different purposes, and people have diverse intentions to experience the connection they provide. They can provide a bridge between our current experience and the sacred. Oftentimes, rituals involve elements that make "crossing" this bridge easier-- symbols, music, using your body, special clothing, specific smells, certain places, and certain people.

Our childhood Monday ritual to the Holy Spirit involved these kinds of elements: a statue of a white dove as a symbol of the Holy Spirit (white symbolized purity, and the dove freedom) with extended wings in overarching encompass. The music we sang surely created special vibrations at which our energy resonated, aiding us to feel connected. Our body free, comfortable, and close to others; our gala uniforms made us feel this day was special. Our decorated patio created a sacred space, and Mother Lupita transmitted serenity and lightness. All these elements in conjunction enabled me to cross the bridge, so that I could feel my humanity and my spirituality together in a vertical sensation of vastness.

Can ritual promote healing? I feel it can actually cause healing. Suffering in need of healing can occur at many levels, not just in the body but also in thoughts, emotions, feelings. All these levels exist at layers of the self below the Spirit. If someone truly accesses the Spirit, the Self may integrate its layers, even if briefly, and curative processes can occur. The person has transcended exclusive identification of the self with these suffering sensations, and so suffering ceases. This brief or long lasting access to the Spirit can be accessed via ritual.

I also believe in more material states of consciousness. For some people, rituals have a purifying purpose such as cleansing and absolving, and in these cases the curative qualities of a ritual are clearer. For example, a man has insulted a friend and is suffering from his actions. He has repented, asked for forgiveness to his friend, and then as part of his Catholic religion, goes to confession and participates in the rite of Eucharist. The ritual itself has now allowed him to release and heal. Or a woman is ill because, according to her cultural beliefs, she is possessed by an angry spirit. A ritual may free her from this possession, and so she will heal.

if I ponder that the very nature of our human existence involves suffering, then I believe a way to end or heal this suffering is to experience the Spiritual, the Self. So even if a ritual is not performed specifically to heal, it still has healing properties for our daily human suffering. Ritual exists in my life quite often. It serves my life to heal, to unite, to pass to a new stage, to find closure, to obtain, to support, to create, to forgive, to forget, to remember. But often it allows me to feel a tiny glimpse of transcendence, to feel for a moment that vertical sensation of safe vastness.

As our day of sun ends, my Micaela, my Silvana, little daughters and myself, free our bodies, wash away the day with water. Our skin and hair still warm and with a cinnamon smell, devotionally we light our candle, and smell our flower oil. Slowly, we kneel towards our rising moon and stars, our heads touching our ground. We feel small . . . we sense the air filling our bodies . . . and leaving it at rest . . . we express gratitude for the love we have, and the pleasures of our lives. As with the Holy Spirit ritual, even if it is just for a moment, the world stops. I feel an immense peace, and everything feels in order and utterly safe. It feels sacred.

Our house remains the same, our breathing is still present, we are all in our places. But now we are all connected through something "greater", something "outside." At the same time we are extremely present "inside." I feel my heart pounding and my blood moving. We stand, we smile at each other, blow out our candle, lie down . . . and let go to sleep.

LETTER TO GEORGE BUCHNER

MICHAEL McCLURE

George Büchner is author of Wozzeck, Danton's Death and other plays and writings. He died in exile at the age of 24 years in 1837 — a fighter for political and spiritual freedom.

Dear George,

I've just finished reading your short story about Lenz the mad playwright and "ape of Goethe." How much I felt it! How much I felt the story! I have been through a madness like Lenz's — but mine was not so pathological as his. I was without Lenz's fear of the dark and his more irrational fears and compulsions. I, too, was in my own Hell of the inert and cold.

I almost could not finish your tale. My old fear began to seep down on me as I read of Lenz. I pushed the fear back and continued the story and knew that I was completely well . . . I was able to drive it all back and continue.

I have just returned to society — that is what I write to tell you.

My return started this way — I ceased to acknowledge the demands of society. I quit fighting against the compulsions and repressions for an instant. The barricade made by my resentment against demands was breached when I ceased to force back rage — a clarity of myself and my life poured out of hidden corners. Now I shalll be a man of life and action! My hermetic life and retirement are over! — It was not quite that easy! —

The horror and the major fears I had are gone, and I return to society!

How stupid I am that I fumble here and repeat. But I do return! And I do not accept what I find on my return. The world is not hopeless and I do not damn it and pull back within myself to a dream of complete destruction and another universe. That is where I have been — in a dream of destruction, held by the sight of a universe I invented and populated with rapine and terror and pale spinning wolves, cold flames, and the pomposity of spirit's aggrandizement. But not now — I am done with that!

I have come back through myself not to a society that is worthless but one that is poisoned. I won't, now that I am here, condone the poisons. You did not pardon them and I will not either. The evils around are not to be fled from but argued against with real flesh bodies.---I've never been here as intensely as I am now.

Wait, yes, I was here this strongly when I was twelve years old and before that. Gradually I retreated year by year, act by act, from the faces of men and women. I did not challenge what I disliked. I weakened and let myself be driven from what I loved! Always within me was a coal of boldness and clear sight of reality, always I could depend on it, but the ember lived without nourishing. I was lucky that it didn't expire. I did not develop the coal — I depended on it.

Suddenly, five days ago I realized that I am twelve years old again! Now I may begin to grow to manhood and with no loss but a gain of extra years that I spent in the strange, and evermore strange, foreign place I inhabited. Now I'm free. Now I'll bring the kernel to full being.

Let me tell you the last things that happened to me in coming back.

I spent two months keeping an intensive journal of all my thoughts and actions and sexuality. I wrote down each petty or important thought and act. Gradually I saw into myself and the simplicity of the hang-ups I live by. Slowly in those two months I beat down the last stages of the blankness that lay on my mind and numbed my actions. I came alive and moved in a larger state than I knew before.

While I worked my deepest fears arose for long moments — I was terrified and made speechless by the look of all living things. When I could not speak I forced myself to make words. I guarded each waking moment to keep myself in motion and activities. If I could not speak when I confronted fear-causing things, then I wrote down in garbled words what I couldn't say aloud. Later I looked at what I wrote to understand the fear and face it better next time.

I burned almost two years of my poetry because it had the stark face and stare of my fear upon it. I couldn't live with it in my sight. I burned all of my writing for the two last and most ugly years except the few pieces that were an outward call from my life. This is it simply. It was right.

I came out able to act, but I was still alone, still cool, and still in a state of drabness. I occupied myself, but I lived in disinterest. Before I battled constantly to keep off madness and fear of it — much of my energy had been cynical and I condemned all that I could. Now I was without negative energy, the Hell that had been my motivation and reason for living.

I spent a few weeks in that new drab state. I kept myself busy so I would not feel it intensely. I kept hoping for something more and better — then a new tension I hadn't felt before came over me. I lay alone in my sleeping bag before the fireplace. I coiled and uncoiled in my body and spirit. I did not think — or if I did think, it was of an anguish I could not identify. I stared about at empty walls, not wanting to stop the releases I felt. Gradually I realized I was being reborn. I did not know what or how, and I did not care except to know it was a rebirth. Somehow I had sureness that I would come to life.

When that stopped I knew something more was coming and I waited. I did not know what was to happen — but I felt better.

In the evenings a feeling of beauty and vibrant clarity and simplicity came over me — the feeling resolved into visions or hallucinations of sweet love-creatures in the air about me. I saw with double sight: I saw what lay before my eyes in the half-dark rooms, and at the same time I looked into crevices of my imagination. In the chasms floated sweet faced creatures of love smiling to me. They were microscopic beasts of no-size and at the same time they were large before my eyes.

They had white, looming, and soft faces and gentle bodies with scales and feathers. They had huge dark eyes, and they sent love to me. They were innocent combinations of tiny eagle and tapeworm and rat and deer. I could see them clearly but could not call them to being at will. They were both a feeling and a sight. I began to change within, to feel love, and to be loved by their simplicity. It was almost nothing.

One evening I drew realizations of the beings— and I wrote the words coming from them. I did not hear them speak the words — but I added them to approximate in some way what the creatures were or meant. The silliness of the words and drawing deserves no apology — I was happy to draw them as I could.

After that night new life came to me. My thoughts were straighter than before. I started a new journal and it was not one of condemnation and self-attack. It was a construction of thoughts and acts that I investigated.

I thought I would die before now and leave one small book of poems. Now I find I have youth and strength and desire to help and make positive action.

I awoke five days ago early in the morning wanting to write my declaration to mankind. I don't know at what instant I accepted the existence of the society about me instead of the inner one that I had made — but I shall stay here where I am now!

So with that realization I write this letter to you.

I believe in the majestic beauty of man and I believe in the simplicity that my senses give evidence of. I believe in a fight for the good that I see and I believe in a condemnation of what is bad for life and mankind. I had retreated from the consciousness of the pains and miseries of others and from the sight of injustice. I had invented reasons (or used my weakness as excuse) not to aid when I could. I had not seen through my prejudices . . . Now, wherever possible, I will put an end to that.

I think the fact that I finally came through with such ease and by such a simple path proves something. I have no declaration to make — except that I shall seek a declaration of good and push to put it into practice. A new era is at hand and it must be joyfully struggled for in full awareness and enjoyment of life. The change is not only inside of myself. In all men there is a new consciousness. A new combat for freedom and happiness and pleasure is beginning every where — I see signs of it in the continents and peoples of the earth. An end can be put to hunger and useless death. I see how many forebearers of this newness lie in the past and history. I see it is a constant struggle, and also merely a fresh budding of what is constant.

I have newly dedicated myself to highest poetry and truth without prejudice.

I hope this reaches you through the trails and swirls of time.

Your friend, Michael

From Meat Science Essays, City Lights Books, 1966.

A Terrible Beauty: For Brad Will

STARHAWK ▮

October 31, 2006

It's the night before the Spiral Dance, our community's annual huge celebration for Samhain, more generally known as Halloween, the ancient feast of the ancestors and honoring of the Beloved Dead, which long predates the Christian feast of All Souls. The Spiral Dance is the biggest, most elaborate ritual our community, Reclaiming the year with intricate altars, a full chorus, dancers, singers, acrobats doing aerial invocations, and a spiral that might include a thousand people. Into all this, we weave some deep magic, both personal and broader than personal, involving the mystery at the heart of our spirituality—death and regeneration.

Each year I take on different roles. Some years I lead the trance, other years I might simply invoke the spirits of the land or play the drum and leave the 'bigger' roles to others. This year my role seems to involve carrying a lot of heavy objects and buckets of sand, building altars and decorating the front of the house. Or not so much actually building and decorating, as providing the materials and suggestions for others to do the creative part.

And this year I'm calling the Dead. So I've been thinking a lot about death, and singing the song we will use to sing the Dead over into a place of renewal. Just before bed, I check my email, and learn that a young man has died, shot to death in Oaxaca where he has gone to cover the teachers' strike and the people's insurrection for Indymedia. His name is Brad Will. I stare at his picture, trying to remember if I know him from all the demonstrations and mobilizations and meetings we have undoubtedly been at together.

In Miami, my friend Andy reminds me. After a wild ritual collaboration between the Pagan cluster and the black bloc, a young man stepped forward with a guitar and began singing Desert Rat's song about Seattle, "When the Tear Gas Fills the Sky." That was Brad—alive, singing, defiant. "I will wash the pepper from your face, and go with you to jail, And if you don't make it through this fight, I swear I'll tell your tale..."

I didn't know him well, but I know so many like him—mostly but not all young, sitting in long meetings in warehouses or donning respirators to gut flood-ruined houses in New Orleans, standing shoulder to shoulder as the riot cops advance, or as the bulldozer moves forward to destroy a home in Gaza. Filing stories at midnight on electronic networks set up by young geniuses with duct tape and component parts in dusty, third world towns, eating cold pasta out of old yogurt tops and sleeping on floors. Hitching rides into war zones and crossing borders. It's as if a whole cohort of souls had arrived on this planet imbued with the unquestioned faith that they were put here to somehow make a difference, to interfere with injustice, to witness, to change the world. Ragged, intemperate, opinionated, passionate, and above all, alive.

And now another one of the tribe is dead, shot down in Oaxaca where a five-month teachers' strike became a full-blown insurrection, the kind that radicals dream of, with streets full of barricades and ordinary people rising up against a rigged election and a corrupt, dictatorial governor. It wasn't much reported in the U.S. papers. But Brad Will was there, with camera and computer, to be a set of eyes.

Now his eyes are closed, forever. I put his name on our list of the Dead. At the Spiral Dance, I see someone has set up a shrine to him on our North altar, where the dead are honored. I meet another activist friend there, who tells me how he remembers Brad: running into a barrage of sound bombs in a demonstration in some foreign city. "I couldn't explain to people that they were harmless," he'd said. "We didn't speak the same language. So I had to show them."

I didn't know him well, but I know how it is to walk into a situation that is dangerous, even life-threatening, how it feels to weigh the risks, to accept them, to tell yourself that you can be at peace with any consequence, and then to walk out into the street in the firm if unconscious belief that you will be lucky that day, once again. I can only imagine how it feels when the bullets rip through flesh, and your severed spirit stares back at a broken body, and in a blaze of light a different journey begins.

We Pagans have no dogma, no official Book of the Dead to outline the soul's journey. If we share any belief in common, it is simply this: that death is part of a cycle that includes regeneration and renewal. That just as the falling leaves decay to fertilize the roots of trees, each death feeds some rebirth.

Death transforms us. The tribe of world-changers has its list of martyrs—the short list of those who are known in the first world—Carlo Giuliani, Huang Hai Lee, Rachel Corrie, Tom Hurndall—and the much longer list of names in some other language—Spanish, indigenous, Arabic, and so many others--who die every day. And the world's religions each have their concept of that transformation, for those whose death is somehow special, powerful and meaningful: martyrs, saints, boddhisatvas. We Pagans don't like to glorify martyrs, but we know that 'sacrifice' means 'to make sacred.' In an instant, that ordinary comrade you remember singing at the fire or arguing at the meeting, someone you might have been charmed or irritated by or attracted to, or not, someone who showed no mark of doom or prescience of what was to come, becomes uplifted into another realm, part symbol, part victim, locus of our deepest love and rage.

William Butler Yeats expressed it best, writing about the Easter Rising in Ireland in 1916, the friends he admired and the ones he disliked, shot by the British.

Being certain that they and I
But lived where motley is worn,

All changed, changed utterly,
A terrible beauty is born . . .

And death transforms the living. When someone close to us dies, we become someone else. When my father died when I was just five years old, my mother was transformed from a beloved wife to a grieving widow. I changed, overnight, from a blessed, fortunate child to someone set apart, marked by a tragedy, missing something deeply important that other children had.

And so one day you are someone with a job and a family and a neighborhood in which you and your kin have lived for generations—and a day later the waters rise and you are homeless, a refugee in a strange place dependent on the kindness of strangers. One day you are a mother filled with hopes and dreams and pride, and the next day you are bereft, with a gaping hole in your heart that can never be filled.

Yet we, the living, have some choice in how we respond to death, and what transformation we undergo. My mother, out of her grief, became a counselor, a therapist, an expert in loss and grieving. Cindy Sheehan, out of her grief for her son Casey, killed in Iraq, became a woman on fire, a modern prophet calling the powerful to justice, who galvanized the movement against the war. Mesha Monge-Irizarry, mother of Idriss Stelley who was shot dead in the Metreon by the San Francisco police, became an advocate for all the victims of police violence. Rachel Corrie's parents took up the cause of justice for the people of Palestine. Grief can open the heart to courage and compassion; rage can move us to action. Out of loss comes regeneration: a terrible beauty is born.

Two Poems Of Enactment

Gary Snyder

One Thousand Cranes

When Carole had cancer prognosis some years back, several of her relatives got together and started folding the little origami called "cranes. They made one thousand paper cranes in different colors and sent them to us, it's a loving custom, to help one get well. Carole got better, thought not cured, and now they hang on swooping strings like flowers on a wall in the house.

In East Asia cranes are noble birds of good fortune, suggesting long life, health, good luck, and troth. They are much in art. Most of the cranes of the world are now centered in Siberia and East Asia—they summer in the north, and winter in north India, eastern China, central Korea, and Japan's big south island, Kyushu.

There are two crane species in North America. One is the endangered whooping crane and the other the gray-beige sandhill crane. One group of sandhill cranes comes down to the Great Central Valley of California: an estimated 30,000 winter over in the area around Lodi, Cosumnes, Thornton, and west toward Walnut Grove. In late February I went with a friend to Cosumnes to look at the flocks of waterfowl one more time before they went back north. We found a place of flooded ricefields full of swimming white-fronted geese, ring-necked ducks, old squaws, teals, coots, and a few tundra swans. And then looking beyond them to a far levee there were rows of cranes pacing, eating, doing their leaping and bowing dance. "Staging up to go back north," they say.

A month later Carole and I were in Berkeley down on 4th Street where we saw an Asian Crafts store called "One Thousand Cranes." It had that subtle incense and hinoki-wood aroma of old Japan. I asked the handsome Japanese woman "How do you say one thousand cranes?" She laughed and said "senbazuru." "Oh yes; one thousand wings of tsuru, cranes." And I told her that my wife and I lived in the Sierra Nevada and watch the cranes flying directly over our place. I remembered back to early March – Carole had been outside, I was in the shop. We began to hear the echoing crane calls. We saw a V – a V made of sub-Vs, flying northeast. They were way high but I did a count of a subsection and it came to eighty birds. They kept coming, echelon after echelon – the cranes just specks, but the echoing calls are loud. More grand flying wedges all afternoon – at least a thousand cranes.

So I told the lady of the store, "Not long ago we watched the cranes go over heading north. They came by all afternoon, at least a thousand." The woman smiled. "Of course. Real life cranes. Good luck for all of us, good luck for you."

From the shady toolshed
hear those "gr r u gr u u g rr ruu"
calls from the sky
step out and squint at the bright
     nothing in sight
just odd far calls
echoing, faint,
grus Canadensis
heading north
       one mile high

THE GREAT BELL OF THE GION

"The great bell of the Gion Temple reverberates into every human heart to wake us to the fact that all is impermanent and fleeting. The withered flowers of the sâla trees by Shakyamuni's deathbed remind us that even those flourishing with wealth and power will soon pass away. The life of fame and pride is as ephemeral as a springtime dream. The courageous and aggressive person too will vanish like a swirl of dust in the wind."

- The Heike Monogatari, 12th century

Heading back to our little house in Murasakino from the Gion Shrine on New Year's eve, with a glowing wick handout from a priest – lit in the New Year sacred fire started anew by bow drill, purified. Walking and lightly swinging the long wick to keep it aglow, in a crowd of people whirling wicks and heading home, finally catch a taxi. Once home start a propane gasplate from the almost-gone wick. Now, a sacred fire in the house. The Gion's huge bell still ringing in the new year: as soft, as loud, at the house three kilometers away as it was at the temple.

Up along the Kamo River
northwest to higher ground.
After midnight New Year's eve:
the great bell of the Gion
one hundred eight times
deeply booms through town.
From across the valley
it's a dark whisper
echoing in your liver,
mending your
      fragile heart.

(Gion Park, Shrine, & Temple in Eastern Kyoto,
named for the park, monastery, and bell of Jetavana in India,
south of Shravasti, where the Buddha sometimes thought)

Day of the Dead Altarmaking: Satisfying for the Soul

Regina Marchi

I loved my grandmother more than I loved anyone. She was my best friend and my biggest fan. As a child, I spent hours with her, baking, sewing, and playing with her vast collection of costume jewelry, stored in a gold rectangular cookie tin with a carnation motif. Each and every time we got together, we would have "tea parties" with cookies, chocolates, and Red Rose tea served creamy white with plenty of milk and sugar. Red Rose was the best tea, Nana said, because it came from Canada, and the Canadians, after all, being members of the British Commonwealth, knew good tea. As an adult, I visited my grandmother every day after work for our ritual tea parties. And when she became too ill to hustle around her kitchen preparing tea for us, I hustled around her kitchen preparing tea for us, as solicitous of her as she had always been of me.

When she passed away in 1996, I was traveling in a remote part of Latin America, with no access to phone or Internet. Unknowing I returned to the US at two o'clock in the morning after an arduous day of air travel, quietly groping my way in the dark of our family home so as not to wake anyone. I noticed the sweet, pungent smell of lilies and, in the thin rays of streetlight that striped the dining room, I recognized the outline of a gigantic arrangement of flowers on the table. Why were they there? With the first seconds of panic tightening my chest, I flipped on the lights to find numerous wreaths of lilies, roses, and mums throughout the living and dining rooms, condolence notes attached. Nana had died a week earlier and was, at that moment, lying somewhere under layers of dank soil. We would never have another tea party. I would never hold her hand again. I would never have a chance to say good-bye.

Years passed and I moved across the country, far from the surroundings of my grandmother. I got a doctoral degree in communication, studying, among other things, Latin American Day of the Dead celebrations and their transformation in the United States. My research examined how these rituals had gone from a primarily religious context in Latin America to a primarily secular one in the United States, becoming alternative media formats for communicating about Latino identity and politics. Yet, I realized that these "invented traditions" (newly adopted rituals designed to establish group cohesion and identity), which took off in the United States in 1972, were much more than mere public assertions of ethnic identity or political commentary. As methods of emotional healing that reached beyond the Latino community to mainstream America, they offer opportunity to process the death of loved ones as well as a response to the loss of community that has come a hallmark of contemporary U.S. society.

Celebrations to honor the dead have been held for thousands of years by peoples around the world. Among the Indigenous agrarian communities of Mexico, Guatemala, Ecuador, Bolivia, Peru, and elsewhere, the fertility of the land, the fertility of family reproduction, and the success of the entire community depend upon paying proper respects to the deceased. In this worldview, the living and the dead are connected forever in reciprocal relationships, and spirits have the ability to intervene in the lives of earthly relatives, helping them to achieve health and prosperity.

For many Indigenous peoples of the Americas, ritual remembrance days are joyous times of family reunion-- liminal periods when relatives, living and dead, temporarily share the same physical space. Heavenly souls visit their earthly kin at these times, and abundant foodstuffs, beverages, flowers, incense, and candles are lovingly prepared and displayed on specially constructed home altars, known in Spanish as "ofrendas" or "offerings." Historically, these celebrations have occurred at harvest times to ensure the availability of copious varieties of flowers, fruits, vegetables, grains, legumes, cacao and other valuable products. The abundance of offerings placed on the altars symbolizes "life" and "vitality" even as the reality of death is acknowledged; life and death are considered part of a continuous cycle in which death begets and supports new life.

When Spanish missionaries arrived in "the New World," they violently imposed Christianity on the various Indigenous peoples of the Americas, attempting to eradicate their pre-existing spiritual practices. Yet, so important and deeply ingrained in native belief systems were rituals for honoring the dead, that missionaries were unable to obliterate them.

While many Latin Americans, being predominantly Catholic, observe All Saints' Day and All Souls' Day in one way or another (i.e. going to church, praying, or leaving flowers by family gravesites), the elaborate rituals I describe here are the particular observances of Indigenous peoples such as the Mixtecs and Zapotecs of Mexico; the Maya of Central America and Mexico; the Quechua and Aymara of South America; and others.

For centuries, Day of the Dead rituals were looked down upon by Latin America's middle and upper classes-- dismissed as the pagan superstitions of "primitives" who refused to modernize. But by the early 1970s, attitudes began to change. This was a period when racial minority groups in the US were attempting to learn about and reclaim their languages, clothing, art, music, rituals and other ancestral traditions that had been lost in processes of slavery, colonization, reservation systems, and forced assimilation. These cultural movements went hand in hand with political movements such as the Women's Movement, the American Indian Movement, Civil Rights Movements, and the Chicano Movement, demanding equal rights for historically disenfranchised populations.

Before the 1970s, most Mexican Americans observed November 1 and 2 (as did Catholics around the world) by attending Mass, having a special family meal, and/or placing flowers at family graves. The elaborate, harvest-themed altar making traditions of southern Mexico's Indigenous cultures were virtually unknown to Mexican Americans, most of whom had lived in the United States for generations. But as young Mexican American artists visited Mexico and learned about Indigenous Day of the Dead traditions, they brought them to the barrios of Los Angeles, San Francisco, Sacramento and elsewhere in the US, where "altar installations" were showcased. In their new context, these public altars were art forms dedicated to teaching about Latin American cultural practices in a Eurocentric, often racist, society.

Since the 1970s, Día de los Muertos exhibits have become annual autumn rituals across the United States. Thanks to the cultural and political work of Latino artists and educators, as well as a growing openness in US society towards non-Western spiritualities and traditions, altar making in remembrance of deceased loved ones is increasingly embraced by a broad spectrum of Latinos and non-Latinos alike.

What attracts them to this ritual? In a society famed for its rugged individualism, contemporary Americans find themselves longing for emotionally satisfying community-building experiences to offset feelings of isolation. During funerary rituals of the pre-industrial United States, mourning individuals were supported by a large community of their extended family, friends and neighbors who lived nearby and knew how to ameliorate the void left by the demise of a loved one. Active rituals of story telling and reminiscing were part of home-centered commemoratory practices that could last all night long or even for multiple days. The hours of collective story telling and even joking about the deceased helped publicly recall his/her contributions to the community, easing the sadness of family members by keeping the person's memory alive. Ritual remembrance days in many non-Western cultures still do this in a way that US Memorial Day-- the official US holiday for visiting cemeteries-- does not.

The somber tone of contemporary Memorial Day observances stands in stark contrast to the vivid ambiance of Day of the Dead, where altars brim with flowers, fruits, and other colorful symbols of life. The growing popularity of Day of the Dead in the United States, frequently referred to in newspapers as "America's newest fall holiday," indicates that mainstream America longs for a medium through which to express repressed emotions regarding death. Regardless of their ethnic, racial or religious backgrounds, people who adopt Day of the Dead altar making traditions express enthusiasm for the opportunity to process feelings about deceased loved ones. As a third generation Japanese American in her mid twenties notes, "It meets a human need for affiliation, on a really elemental level." A middle aged Anglo-American states, "There is no venue in American tradition which lets us honor and celebrate our dead. Once people have died, their memory becomes a private matter for the family. There is no public remembrance past the funeral. It's as if they were swept under the carpet and we move on to the next thing. With Día de los Muertos, the entire community is involved in a public acknowledgment of the dead."

Repeatedly, people I interview tell me that making Day of the Dead altars helps them heal spiritually from the physical loss of someone they loved. They describe a dichotomy between "U.S." ways of relating to death, which they consider "unfulfilling" or "lonely," and Day of the Dead rituals, which they call "celebratory," and "supportive." Today, communal altar making events during Day of the Dead season have become popular in locations ranging from substance abuse rehabilitation facilities to non-denominational religious organizations, to violence prevention organizations, classrooms, museums, and community centers, where both individual and collective altars are erected in memory of a community's deceased. Participants typically bring photos, stories, and favorite mementos of departed loved ones to share. They place on the altar candles, photos, books, musical albums, jewelry, articles of clothing, crocheted doilies, alcoholic beverages, cigars or any other items that "speak" of the lives of the departed. Participants are often invited to make a variety of decorations for the altar and/or write personalized messages to the deceased on index cards to be placed on the altar. Adorned with colorful woven cloth, photos, fruits, breads, cookies, tamales, hot chocolate, flowers, art work, and other "offerings," the altars ultimately present a visual, olfactory, and sometimes even musical panoply of life experiences and memories that connect the living with the dead. Each person who helps create the altar (and sometimes bystanders) may stand and speak about a person s/he is remembering.

For many, creating a Day of the Dead altar may be the first opportunity they've ever had to speak publicly about a deceased loved one, regardless of how many years have elapsed since the death. The atmosphere is both happy and emotional, as people recall stories about their deceased friends and family, sharing lessons learned from them, and discussing attributes they most loved about them. Yet, it also opens up new possibilities for connectedness and realizations that the dead are always with us, if we keep them alive in our thoughts and conversations. As rituals, these activities satisfy spiritual and emotional needs, strengthen social bonds, and offer forms of collective education.

When we share stories about people who have touched our lives deeply, we also share a part of our own life story. In the process, we realize how strongly certain aspects of the deceased live on within us, and are able to convey those aspects to others. A visual arts professor who has participated in Day of the Dead altar exhibits on his university campus states: "For students who aren't of Mexican ancestry, and even for those who are, it gives them an opportunity to connect with their own personal history, and that's a spiritual resource that we're often denied." Connecting with those who have gone before us can help mend lives torn by heartbreak. Day of the Dead altar making has been effective in inner city schools, where populations are disproportionately affected by adversity, helping students to express their feelings in a supportive environment and remember, in a positive way, family members lost to domestic violence, gun violence, gang violence, drugs, or war.

Even in museum and art gallery settings, Day of the Dead altars can help people to heal. An example is the Oakland Museum of California, where artists and local residents have created Day of the Dead altar installations annually since 1994. Each year, some 20,000 people attend the museum's six-week exhibit, making it the best-attended show in the museum's calendar. The chief curator of education believes the exposition's popularity is the opportunity it provides for people to reflect upon and talk about death: "A number of people have said that they don't have anything from their culture that helps them deal with death . . . We've had a number of grief counselors and people from the health profession who have come here and used this exhibit with their clients to help them process death." Another employee added, "We've received lots of letters from people thanking us and saying that it's helped them reflect, or telling us how they've adopted the tradition. Not just Latino people. One of the great things we have here is a wall of reflection, where you can write messages to people who have passed on. I've seen families crying, hugging each other. So there's something we can offer people who are in pain, to help them heal."

After studying Day of the Dead as a social scientist for the better part of a decade, I decided to make my own Day of the Dead altar in 2007. On the eve of November 1, I invited a group of family and friends to my home, asking them to bring mementos of their deceased loved ones. Earlier that day, I visited several Latino bakeries and flower shops to acquire bunches of marigolds and special pan de muerto, the "bread of the dead" popular in Mexico. I invited my nieces and nephews, ranging in age from three to nine, to join me that afternoon in creating altar decorations of paper flowers, papel picado (intricate crepe paper cutouts used in Latin America to decorate for parties) and "lanterns" (made of discarded 2-liter plastic soda bottles covered in colorful tissue paper with mini votive candles placed inside).

Going to the oldest piece of furniture I own, an antique cedar trunk where I store special clothing, photos, and other items that are precious to me, I began to open up various boxes carefully stacked inside. I found a tiny heart-shaped gold locket belonging to my grandmother, with fading photos of her and my grandfather placed inside. I found beautiful hand sewn silk undergarments, slightly brittle now with time, that were part of my great grandmother's marriage trousseau. I spent a long time looking at old photos of my grandparents, remembering happy moments together, as well as photos of my great grandparents whom I'd never met, recalling all I had learned about them from my grandmother. I even found the rectangular cookie tin with the carnation motif, filled to the brim with costume jewelry. When I opened it, the familiar perfumed scent of my grandmother's house came to me, still lingering inside the box after so many years.

Before my guests arrived, I began putting together a three-tiered altar – a style common in areas of southern Mexico. First, I covered the dining room table (the largest and middle level of the altar) with beautiful tapestries I had acquired in my travels to Guatemala, Ecuador, Africa and elsewhere. Then, I moved the cedar trunk in front of the table, also covering it with tapestries, to create a lower level for the altar. The highest level of the altar was a wooden fruit-packing crate I found in the trash, placed on top of the table and covered with colorful woven fabric. On the highest level of the altar, I placed large photos of my grandparents – my grandmother smiling like one of the Andrew Sisters in her 1940s updo, my grandfather handsome and strong in his merchant marine uniform. On the lower levels, I placed the gold locket, the tin box of jewelry, my grandmother's favorite Engelbert Humperdinck album, and a steaming cup of freshly brewed Red Rose tea. I also added my grandfather's reading glasses (he had quit high school to earn money and help his family during the Great Depression, but remained a voracious reader his entire life); some jewelry he made for me when he took up the hobby of silversmithing during his retirement (his father had been a silver smith); and some of his favorite pecan pralines from New Orleans (his home town).

At 8:00 pm, my invited friends and family arrived. The children excitedly placed the lanterns and flowers on the various levels of the altar, while the adults lit the candles and created an "arch" of bent corn stalks from my garden, affixed to the top of the altar. (It is said that the spirits like an archway through which to enter.) From the arch, we hung apples, pears, and bananas, attaching strings to the fruit stems and tying them to the arch, in a decorative style common in altars created by Mexico's Mixtec people. Each person placed photos of loved ones on the altar, along with mementos, and told us about the meanings these people and items had for them. A friend from Turkey brought a photo of the beloved nursemaid from her childhood, with whom, she explained, she had spent more time and felt closer to than her own parents. She placed it on the altar along with a traditional Turkish headscarf worn by rural Turkish women and some "Turkish delight" candies. A friend from Mexico brought a photo of her father, a bottle of his favorite beer, and some tamales. She shared with us that her father had fought as a child in the Mexican Revolution alongside Pancho Villa. An Irish friend tried her hand at baking pan de muerto from a recipe she found on the Internet, placing it on the altar. My sister brought the pink and green blanket that our grandmother had knit for her when she was born, folding it neatly on the altar as she explained how her own child now loved it the way she once did. My brother brought my grandfather's harmonica, which he had inherited, and a package of those sticky chocolate cupcakes covered in pink marshmallow and shredded coconut that Grandpa used to enjoy. My uncle, who is originally from Venice, Italy, placed a photo on the altar of his mother standing in the Piazza San Marco. She had died in a car accident when he was only 15, so none of us had ever met her. He almost never spoke of his parents, but took this opportunity to share memories about them.

As the circle of family and friends added items to the altar, it grew more complex and beautiful. All of us were as wide eyed as my young nieces and nephews, listening to the stories each person told about the items they brought and the person they were remembering. My mother and aunt shared stories about our deceased relatives that I had never heard. My friends, who hailed from different countries, races, and religions, shared aspects of themselves that I might not otherwise have had an opportunity to learn. And, for the first time in many years, I felt that we were all together again as a family, my grandparents sitting in the room with us, just as they always used to do at family holidays.

Everyone enjoyed the evening, thanking me profusely for organizing it. Even certain relatives who commented beforehand that they thought it was a "weird" thing to do ended up being really moved, and asked if we could do it again the following year. The altar was so splendid that I left it up for several days. Word spread among my extended family, friends and neighbors, and people dropped by my house over the next couple of days to look at it or take photos. Even my 18-year old cousin, too busy and too cool to hang out with spirits on November 1, brought a group of his friends to see the altar the next day.

Now I create a Day of the Dead altar each fall. My family has enthusi-astically adopted it as a new holiday ritual that helps shed light, especially for the children, on some of the original intentions of Halloween or "the Hallowed Eve." And my grandmother, I'm sure, looks forward to sharing a cup of Red Rose tea with the family every year. She would be terribly disappointed, now, if we stopped.

HAND-MADE BINOCULARS: VISION AS RITUAL AND HEALING

J. REBECCA BUSBY

AT AGE 5 I RECALL GETTING OUT OF MY FATHER'S NEW 1957 RED BUICK. I slid across the clear plastic seat cover that had a pattern of tiny silver stars, and out the door I went. I was dressed in a new white dress with fuzzy red hearts all over and my best black patent-leather shoes. I stood with my brother, who was 9, in front of a huge Tudor style house adjacent to two more just like it on a semi-circle driveway surrounded by acres of azaleas. I was met by a tall, thin, and lovely lady named Mrs. Harrell.

I don't recall the conversation; I probably didn't hear much except for the words, which implied that I was now going to be living at what turned out to be an orphanage. At that I slid into a ritual action; I covered my eyes by encircling them with my hands shaped like a small pair of binoculars. I am told I walked around this way for several weeks. I don't recall the time frame, but I do recall the comfort of having a means to regulate what I took in visually. For a child with little power or control in a situation, I see this as an innately protective and wise behavior.

Try it. Hold your hands up like binoculars and look at the world around you. You can narrow or expand your "Vision." You can look up, down, sideways. You can even close off all vision. As humans we utilize vision external and internal. Vision is integral to growth, achievement and dreams. I look out on the world and see daily mundane life, but I sometimes see the possible or the dream. Internally I see memories, but I also see my hopes and dreams. Vision has been one of the keys to my life path and to my spiritual awaking. Many years later I realize my hand-made binoculars were the first of many re-enactments in which I experienced of the myth of Inanna descending to the underworld.

I began a path of spiritual introduction in that orphanage, which was a lovely, warm, and wonderful place, by the way. Located in Mobile, Alabama, the Wilmer Hall Episcopal Children's Home, as it is now called, was begun in 1864 to take in orphans of the Civil War; 145 years later, it still continues to do exceptional work. I lived there five years, returning to live with my Mother at age ten.

The split of my family followed my mother falling into a depression after the death of her father. At that time in 1957 it was unusual for fathers to take the full responsibility of raising children. My father took my brother and me to live in Mobile, which was 200 miles from my Grandparents' home where we had been living. His intent was to place us in boarding schools, but I was too young. He then made the decision to keep us together and placed us in the orphanage. He and my mother visited regularly, but a divorce followed the breakup of the family, and custody was not settled for five years.

The transition to the orphanage must have been a tremendous rip in the fabric of our lives. However, I do not recall this. I do recall longing for my family and for the comfort of my grandparents' home. This change was both a death/birth in my life. To lose such comfort and love as we had in our grandparents' home was certainly unlike anything this five year old had ever felt. However, it was a birth as well. What came from the orphanage was a different way of life-- exposure to living with 60 children ages 5-18 years of age and house parents who truly cared for us. Becoming a part of the Episcopal Church was a very different style of life. My grandparents owned two acres of land so we grew our food and had many animals. Wilmer Hall was located in an upper class neighborhood. The buildings of the orphanage were grand compared to my grandparents' simple home, but Wilmer Hall never fulfilled the loss I felt. I began searching for understanding even at the age of five or six.

As I grew up, I continued searching; I visited virtually every religious faith possible in a quest for knowledge, understanding, and a place of worship that felt like a spiritual home for me. Even though they all had elements of delight and uniqueness, none felt right. I was after all searching for answers to both psychological issues of loss and a spiritual seeker on a path to some inner Vision I had yet to discover. I settled on Unitarian because of its inclusive, open minded, and intellectually stimulating stance.

In 1979 at age 26 I was diagnosed with Rheumatoid Arthritis (R.A.) and shortly thereafter moved to San Diego. I had been a Computer Systems Analyst for 12 years, but found it stressful, lonely, without the human connection I longed for. I began what had been a life-long Vision-- becoming a clinical psychologist. Vision had guided me through spiritual exploration, mind-body and holistic exploration, geographic change and ultimately to my "daimon", as James Hillman refers to our inward destiny in his book The Soul's Code: In Search of Character and Calling (1996, p. 8). Hillman uses the word daimon interchangeably with destiny to describe the inner spark of who we are meant to become.

A chronic illness is a powerful thing; it has the potential to guide us to many places we may never have sought out, had we been otherwise unaffected. Personally, R.A. certainly has been an amazing teacher, acting simultaneously as a torturer and spiritual guide. For 30 years, I have lived with the uncertainty of R.A., yet in those 30 years I have never lost my Vision. I have gone down to the underworld with Inanna through Goddess Spirituality many times, only to return with treasures and healing indescribable to people who do not live with chronic pain and illness. Rheumatoid arthritis can go into remission, though mine never has. It flares up with a vengeance, and as a result has changed my life by focusing my Vision. Along the way I found my twofold spiritual path -- Goddess Spirituality and clinical psychology.

The myth of Inanna has replayed a role in my life over and over, as it has for many women. The myth of Inanna involves a woman going willingly into the underworld and returning. My Vision required me to become more limited, but also more expansive, but in ways I was not fully conscious of until after the event. Often the ritual is not understood until after the event, and even then we can only process the experience in bits and piece. It may take years to fully understand a ritual.

We enter and leave the world through ritual-- a state of awe accompanies the beginning and the end of life. Along life's way, we also have daily rituals, some of which we are conscious and others not. Although we can choose to be conscious of these rituals, humans are not born as highly conscious beings. Fortunately, events can occur at certain times of our lives that succeed in waking us up to consciousness. These moments may be anywhere on a continuum of sad to joyful, and how we react to these events tells a story. Finally, some of these events may be stepping stones to spiritual awaking.

My personal path turned out to be Goddess Spirituality. My dissertation, Goddess-Focused Spirituality: A Survey of Women's Experiences and Implications for Therapy is the first of its kind in psychology.

What I learned was that I actually had a very small vision of the power that the Goddess has worldwide. I had no idea of the vast numbers of women eager to share their stories and experiences. I know now that these women seek the Goddess as a means of empowerment that this can be used in therapy and/or ritual to heal. My work in psychology, the R. A., and the Goddess empower me daily to dig deep and return to the light, knowing I am growing into my "daimon."

As I look back along this path with my hand-made binoculars, I see both the narrow and the expansive Vision it took get to this point. I see, I feel, I survive, I dive deep to the underworld, I return renewed, I touch and am touched to have made this healing journey many times. I am not cured, but I am "put right" by moments of "sacred action." I am honored to have been contacted by the 5,520 people worldwide who have had their own ritual and healing journey to and through Goddess Spirituality. And I wonder what new and wondrous learning my Goddess binoculars will bring into focus next?

Ride Across California: A Family Ritual

Ron Stolberg

The best things in life often happen when you least expect. That's what I learned from proposing a bike ride with my 10 year old son. Aaron hadn't been on his fancy dust-gathering bike in about a month. The funny thing is, I didn't really want to go on a bike ride. I just needed him to ride his bike so I could practice taking movies with a new HD camera that has an option to mount it on handlebars or bike helmet. I'm kind of a geek about electronic toys like that.

Something else about me is that I am always complaining that my generation and my cultural group don't have traditions, ceremonies, or rituals. In fact, I am terribly jealous of my friends who have strong religious affiliation, who have cultural or ethnic family traditions. And wish I had more in my life.

Now back in the driveway getting ready for a camera-testing excuse of a bike ride, it will end up that Aaron and I experience exactly what I had been craving. We will become part of a tradition that has its very own history and -- to my delight-- its very own rituals.

It's called the Ride Across California or RAC, and we participated in the 21st consecutive ride. It started with a child's question "can I ride my bike across America?" An elementary school principle and one of his teachers had just read Hey Mom, Can I Ride My Bike Across America?: Five Kids Meet their Country by John S. Boettner. They crafted an optimistic plan. They thought that a bike ride across California would be the perfect tool to teach young children that if they have a dream, there is a way to achieve it. If you could ride your bike nearly 300 miles all the way across a big state like California when you were 10 or 11 years old, imagine what you can do when you are 15, or 18, or a grown-up?

A simple request: "Aaron, are we going on a quick bike ride after dinner?" is all it took. As I went to the garage to fit the bikes and helmets with cameras, my son ran up to his room. He arrived in a day-glow yellow riding jersey, skin-tight bike pants, fingerless gloves and a helmet. He said we couldn't go without doing our ABC's. I was in a hurry and a bit frustrated because I wanted the light to be just right. The ABC's didn't even enter my thoughts. But it ends up Aaron was reciting a ritual that I hadn't paid attention to. The ABC's stand for Air, Brakes, and Chain, and he was methodically going over his checklist like a pilot before takeoff.

But this isn't a story about checking to see if there is air in your tire before going on a ride. It is the story of how a community has been working nearly a quarter century to teach 10-year-olds to become self-confident, goal-setting, responsible young people.

In retrospect I had known about the RAC for years. Our street, a cul-de-sac, is home to about 20 families. Over the last decade I have seen no fewer than eight of these families preparing for the ride. The legend begins with stories of campfires and childhood bliss. I heard more than once "that was the best week of my life." They were head deep into a well evolved ritual, handed down for decades from family to family, 5th grader to 5th grader (girls and boys; there might have been more moms riding with their kids than dads).

Learning Our Rituals

Six months before the actual RAC ride, you are told that you and your child will do several hundred miles of training and attend weekly information meetings. These meetings have creative titles like "Rules of the

Road I", and "Rules of the Road II" and... well, you get the picture. At the same time we are given the "Ride Schedule" which outlines what we will be doing nearly every Saturday for the next six months. We rode in the rain, sun, wind . . . and up some really big hills.

While we were practicing our ABC's and putting in miles, each ride had an unexpected obstacle and lesson. Every group has a leader who rides "point" to set the pace, and someone who rides at the back called the "caboose." Our training rides could have 50 or more riders, and in a group that big there will be really fast riders, really slow riders, riders with mechanical problems, and those who have something else go wrong. For the caboose(s), this category includes getting sick, running out of water, wanting to give up, and all sorts of things you can't plan for. We were quickly becoming much more than casual acquaintances and neighbors; we were becoming family. This family had to take care of each other and trust one another with our lives. We were developing the rituals that would keep us safe and help us obtain our goal of riding across California.

So for six months before bed I did my ABC's, laid out my helmet with glasses and gloves, filled a backpack. Each time it became easier, with less thought. Little did I know how important these simple behaviors would become.

The Beginning

Ride Across California travels the short direction across, which is just shy of 300 miles and takes a week. Another name for the ride is River to Riptide because it starts at the Colorado River, at the border between California and Arizona, and goes to the Pacific Ocean in San Diego. Our iteration of the ride consisted of about 180 people—80 or more 5th graders, I heard.

All riders start the first day by placing the back tire of their bikes into the Colorado River. Yuma Arizona is just a few miles over the sand dunes, and the border with Mexico is about 100 yards away. Together Aaron and I place our back tires in the river, just as over a thousand RAC riders have done in the past. And away we go! . . . the first leg an easy 20 miles to

Gold Rock Ranch, with visions of campfires and a good night's sleep.

Away we go, straight into the wind and onto sand-blown trails impassable unless you got off and carry your bike. It took about 10 minutes before I saw my first 5th grader go flying over the handlebars into the sand. We all jumped off our bikes and began to walk along the easy 20 miles in the desert at 90 degrees.

After some hiking and some uphill riding into the wind, the sign said "Welcome to Gold Rock Ranch." If I thought the ride was going to be the hard part, I was mistaken. The part I wasn't prepared for was waiting.

At the end of each day's ride you gather your gear from the support truck. Our gear consisted of two folding chairs, clothes, sleeping bags, air mattresses, bike gear, and some packaged food. Once you have your gear you need to find a place to set up your tent. I was tired and thought I would rest up a bit before making camp. Aaron, being 10 years old, ran off to explore with his friends. Dinner would be served in about an hour; a group campfire would be lit after dark. I found Aaron at dinner, to discover that he would basically reject every prepared meal the rest of the trip.

For our night's accommodations we decided on a plot protected by some bushes and down in a dry river-bed. We had heard that the wind sometimes comes up at night. Aaron and I could set up our small two person low profile pop-up in about 10 minutes, with another 5 minutes for blowing up the air mattresses and unrolling the sleeping bags. At least that's how long it took in our living room. The sun was setting, and the wind had come up to a respectable 20-25 mph. We laid out the tarp where the tent would be set up, and a gust picked it up and blew it down the river-bed. Aaron ran after it, laughing all the way. We decided that heavy rocks would help keep the tarp in place long enough to get the tent set up. The wind became stronger and the tent-making became funnier to Aaron (not so much to me). Eventually, we got it set up, the air mattresses filled, and the sleeping bags out. All that was left was to try to get the kids to go to bed. All day on a bike doesn't really tire them out.

Once we're in the tent, sleep comes easily until the wind really picks up. That first night we got a few hours, but by 1 am I thought the tent was going to blow away with us in it. We were lucky to be in a tent that only stood a few feet high. Several of our friends with stand-up tents had tent posts snap, and they were whipped around pretty good. Things were blown away in the night, some found in the morning stuck in the brush. I would guess that my average night consisted of only a few hours of sleep, but Aaron seemed to sleep and found it all rather amusing and exciting.

THE MIDDLE

The mornings start early. Most families are up at 6 am. The kids want to run around and play. Aaron doesn't like whatever was being served for breakfast. Roll up the sleeping bags, air mattresses, tents. Hope your stuff doesn't blow away. Drink as much water as you can and lather up with sun screen. Finally, drop the gear off at the truck and hit the road by 8 am. Ride all day, stop for pictures and snacks along the way. Marvel at just how big California is, even the short way across.

Repeat seven times.

Riding was the easy part. Not that being on a bike for six to eight hours a day is by any stretch easy, but we trained for that. We looked out for each other's children, and we helped each other along the way. There were flat tires, crashes, lots of tears, 90 degree days and a morning with snow. On the ride we fell back on the strong habits we developed for riding safely as a group. We wore bright colors, obeyed the street signs, and rode with confidence built by hundreds of miles of training. There were pep talks almost daily. Sometimes you gave one, sometimes you got one, it just depended on the day.

Camping, on the other hand, took a little more time to get accustomed to. The first night Aaron and I did everything wrong, but we got our tent up, survived the night, and hit the road in the morning. We learned a lot that first 24 hours. We developed a pattern of behaviors that became more and more efficient. Each night before falling asleep we would laugh about the funny things that happened that day, then in the morning we would laugh about the funny things that happened during the night. Quickly, we developed our rituals that became the backbone of a successful RAC. It went something like this:

Get to camp.
Get your gear.
Hydrate.
Find rocks big enough to hold your tarp down in the wind.
Put up tent, sleeping bags, and air mattress before dark.
Eat and just make sure Aaron finds enough calories for the next day.
Let the kids go play until they can't play anymore.
ABC's, helmet, gloves, glasses, and fill the backpack with snacks spare inner tubes.
Give up trying to get Aaron to change his clothes or get hosed off before bed.
Sleep a few hours.
Pack it all up.
Find a few more calories and ride until you do it all again.

THE END

After about 280 miles and seven days, we reached the coast in Carlsbad. The symbolic finish to the ride occurs when your front tire enters the Pacific Ocean, so we all rode straight for it. Cheering family and friends lined the last few hundred yards. We all felt like we had just won the Tour de France.

Everyone shared in obvious sense of accomplishment. But the more I reflect upon the RAC, the more I see that the sense of community and tradition is what I hold closest. To date untold numbers of kids and parents have gone through the same training rides and evening meetings. They have developed the same road awareness and respect for how diverse and big California is. Most importantly they developed their own rituals that guided them to learn and grow and be recognized. The guideline was, have a big dream and find a way to make that dream come true. The necessary rituals, as Aaron demonstrated to me, are in all of us. You just have to find them.

One last thing. The RAC is a Family Ritual for lots of reasons. There's the family of riders you share the journey with, and the extended family you join upon completion of the ride, knowing that you share the experiences and rituals which will be with you forever. For Aaron and myself there is also the plan that we will be completing the ride again. This time we will be handing down the traditions and value of our extended family and teaching the rituals that kept us safe. This year I will have yet another fifth grade son ride the RAC, and it will truly be a family ritual. I can't wait.

For those interested in learning more about the Ride Across California, the Rancho Family YMCA in San Diego has all the information you need. The following web address is a great place to start: http://www.rancho.ymca.org/test/bike-club-rac.html

A fun video of everyone finishing the ride at the beach can be found on YouTube at:

http://www.youtube.com/watch?v=ZdB-D23AU8I

Finally, credit needs to go to Dennis Bucker and Mike Fickel, child educators who were responsible for the birth of the RAC. Today it rests in the good hands of Gary Rossi and Jesse Pazdernik, two of the most inspiring motivators I have ever met. In conjunction with the Rancho Family YMCA and scores of volunteers, these great people have given over a 1,000 families a sense of accomplishment after dreaming big.

2

PERSONAL HEALING AND RITUAL

Digging My Grave: An Encounter with Mother Earth

Heriberto Hescamilla

Digging our graves took us the better part of the day. The earth we dug into had been used for ritual burials by others so it was fairly soft. But in addition to the digging, we had to haul all of the materials from the storage shed to the grave sites. We also took time for several hikes on the rocky terrain that surrounded the burial grounds. After a few hours of digging, it was impossible to ignore my whiney and complaining lower back. The more I dug, the louder it cried. In my everyday world, I work seated in front of a lap top computer, in what must be the most ergonomically incorrect posture possible. It's also been a few years since I stopped regularly practicing Yoga, but I've made it a habit to do some of the stretches, to jog or walk, and keep a garden. So I am not a complete stranger to physical activity. But the strenuous walks, the digging, and sleeping on the ground brought my physical sensations to the forefront of my awareness, pulling my attention out of the clouds, where it resides most of the time, and into my tired arms, sore back and overloaded legs.

We were situating our graves around a central fire pit. The diameter of the burial site was about 20 to 25 yards. There were only six of us and we were well distributed around the circle, with at least 5 yards between one person and the next. I remember wanting an undisturbed night, so

I deliberately sought as much distance as possible from my companions.

We had each taken a few minutes to find our own "spot." I chose one on the west side of the fire, not through feeling, but reason. I have learned through attending sweat lodge and other Native American ceremonies that the west is the direction of introspection. In various traditions, this direction is associated with the thunderbird, the black bear, darkness, and women. It is the place where the Sun meets Mother Earth after its daily trek across the heavens. I thought facing west would be an appropriate way to spend a night in the ground.

Each one of us shoveled the earth out of our own graves, but we gathered as a group to inspect and add the finishing touches to each. My grave was about 3 feet deep, with 4 to 6 inches of space between my body and each side. The final opening left very little room for movement. The finished rectangular hole measured approximately about 4 feet wide by 6 and half feet long and 3 feet deep.

We constructed the grave's covering with similar attention to detail, also doing most of the work independently, but coming together for the final touches. To seal the grave, we laid slats of wood across the entire opening to the grave. The wooden pieces were about an inch thick and no more than three of four inches wide. The wooden slats were just sturdy enough to support the tarp that completely covered the opening. At the end where our heads would lie, we pulled back the tarp and set aside three or four of the underlying slats; leaving just enough of an opening to crawl into the grave. We finished the grave by shoveling about 6 inches of dirt on to the tarp. The first few shovelfuls of dirt on the tarp resonated eerily from inside the empty grave, like drumbeats. I paused to listen for a few minutes. Then for the last few minutes, my companions and I shoveled to a steady drumbeat of earth falling on the graves.

In the early evening we gathered in a circle around the fire for final preparations. I like the fire's warmth. The smell of smoke fills my head with memories that I should tell you about some day, but not today. The last major task before entering the grave was to confess ourselves. This was not my first confession to Tatewari fire, but it seems that each time, the anticipation causes me more anxiety and apprehension. At this point in my life, the "purpose" of confession has become frustratingly elusive, and at the same time a critical need. Webster's defines confession as the act of "acknowledging or avowing by way of revelation." It is the process of making something that already exists known. This definition gives no association to shame, guilt, pain or suffering. But when asked to confess, those are the images that emerge for me. I suspect that growing up as the oldest boy in a Mexican household, it was impossible for me not to inherit a somewhat bleak attitude toward life and responsibility. And even though I was not heavily indoctrinated into Catholicism, I have always seen confession as speaking out a thought, feeling or behavior that has offended an all-knowing God, its purpose to avoid retribution and punishment.

I suspect that our ancestors saw the act of confession differently, a way of living among companions, and not something one does periodically to a person or deity. My Wirrarika friends tell me that they confess completely and publicly during their ceremonies. From what I gather, it is a central part of their lives. At this point in my life, what makes the most sense is that being "impeccable" (as Castañeda writes) or "without sin" (as the biblical Jesus was often described) means living a life of continual confession, always revealing, transparent or "authentic." The impeccable person expresses life freely, never holding back or holding on. What an expectation!

So what was my confession?

I confessed to making a burden out of the life that people share with me. I confessed to not honoring that creative spark inside of me and inside of others. I judge people and resent them for not living as I believe they should. I assume to know how they should live. I hold on to my words a lot, fearing how others might respond to them. I willfully hold on to the burden that I consciously make out of the life I am granted. I confessed this to Grandfather Fire and to my companions around the circle. My companions each took a turn asking the Grandfather for help in cleaning themselves of the burdens they had created and carried. By the end of the round, I definitely needed and asked for a group hug.

After a few last minute instructions, we walked to the burial sites. I don't recall the exact order of the burials. I believe that Jennifer, to my left and with her feet oriented toward the fire, was first. To her right, we planted Rusty, a close friend that I met at my first retreat. Alexey, the systematic and methodological man from the Ukraine, came next. He and Rusty were oriented toward the north. Joy, another close friend from my first retreat, was next. I recall that her head was toward the center of the site, toward Grandfather Fire. Gloria was next, with her feet pointed toward the South. We gathered as a group to bury each other. As we moved counterclockwise around the circle, the group grew smaller. Victor buried me last.

I carefully stepped into the grave, feet first until they touched the bottom of my old burgundy-colored sleeping bag. I'm not sure what I expected to feel. The thought that I should be afraid crossed my mind. As my head came to rest on the pillow, the smell of dirt and damp air quickly filled my awareness. I calmly accepted that the tarp snuffed out what last threads of light were left by the night. My body responded to the sound of the dirt as it hit the tarp above me. Hearing the dirt drop, from inside the grave, disturbed me even more than it had earlier in the day. "Victor must do that on purpose", I thought to myself, "He throws the dirt on a little harder than necessary for dramatic effect." But I had been on the other side; I'd thrown dirt on my companions so I knew that the dirt was thrown carefully, ceremoniously, covering all possible sources of light. But it sounded very loud and unnerving.

In the darkness I could hear Victor walking around the site. I heard him kneel down over my grave as he assured that the breathing hole behind my head was properly functioning. I heard muffled words of encouragement through the dirt and tarp.

I entered my grave that night with the intention of lying on my back and talking to Mother Earth, just talking without stopping until I could not talk anymore. And since the notion of Mother Earth brings to mind images of growth, of trees and plants, it seemed logical that I should begin with my experience with this aspect of my life. I intended to build my connection with Mother Earth as I had done with Grandfather Fire, by talking about my relationships without stopping, just pouring the words out of my body, "de Corazon" as we say in Spanish. I was not sure what to expect.

I also took a concern into the grave. Sleep has never come easy, and sleep on my back has been impossible for as long as I remember. I can just lie there, not really conscious of any worries, simply unable to sleep. If I focus on relaxing I can sometimes fall asleep, but will inevitably have nightmares and awaken within a few minutes. The nightmares have always been about being chased by what can best be described as an "evil presence." I wanted to use this opportunity to rid myself of this chronic problem. In fact, let me confess a little further, I wanted to face this "evil presence" once and for all and fall asleep peacefully on my back. That was one intention.

As Victor's footsteps faded into the darkness, leaving me with the damp smell of Mother Earth, the first thought to cross my mind was "when do I get out of here?" (In the group discussions that followed, it became evident to me that this has been my very disrespectful attitude toward life. Imagine the unforgivable act of greeting someone and immediately thinking about leaving). I felt anxiety and the fleeting touch of fear.

That night, I simply noted my response without further reflection and set about the task that I had intended. I proceeded to tell Mother Earth everything that came into my awareness. I told her about my first five years in Mexico, growing up the orange groves and cornfields of Nuevo Leon. I told her about the prickly pear spines that my aunt meticulously pulled out of my fingers and palms. I told her about my experience with the land, the hot days, the chicharras, and the smell of wet dirt during the rain. I described what it was like walking alongside my grandfather Gustavo as he cared for the oxen; as his machete cleanly sliced the corn stalks; the crunching sounds the goats made when their teeth slowly ground the yellow shoots. I told Mother Earth of the walks to and from my abuelito's adobe and straw jakal and his cornfields. I described my abuelita's smoke-filled kitchen and watching her grind corn into masa. I told her about leaving this world behind in January of 1958.

My legs were sweating and itchy. I wanted to take off my blue jeans. Unbuckling my belt, I pulled them down as best I could, careful not to brush up against the walls of my grave. The dirt was loose, so any contact would bring little streams of finely ground dirt trickling onto my head or the sleeping bag. I managed to push my jeans into a crumpled ball at my feet. I unzipped my sleeping bag. The air, even as it grew cold, felt good.

I continued my conversation with Mother Earth, telling her about the big pecan tree in our backyard, a tree that suffered through my home made darts, makeshift arrows, sand-filled kicking bags and other expression of childish fantasies. Every fall, the tree's dark gray arms dropped tons of pecans on the grass below. It continued to do so even after Carla's harsh winds amputated half of her limbs. But this monologue was still rehearsed. I had thought about what I wanted to say for much of the day.

I confessed to Mother Earth how I gradually separated myself from the corn, the pecan trees and my mother's geraniums. The words started to drag a little. There are only so many words that one can prepare in advance. Searching for what to say next became a challenge. My heart was not pouring out repressed memories or previously unconscious insights, as I had envisioned. No demons yet. My mind would wander on a regular basis, I wondered about the time. I thought of my wife and children back home. Thoughts of my work and projects also meandered through, sometimes drawing my attention for a few seconds. It's amazing how much goes through our minds, mostly undetected.

I recounted my adolescent years. My attention shifted away from plants and to schoolwork, thinking about girls and watching a lot of television. I continued to talk.

I felt a resurgence of energy as I told the earth about my wife, Yolanda. When I met her in 1978, I had been practicing yoga and meditating regularly. But I wasn't healthy. I was down from my high school weight of 160 to about 98 pounds. In addition to the weight, I had forgotten a lot. I couldn't understand the attention my wife gave her plants. I told Mother Earth about the giant Dieffenbachia, Fiddle Leaf Fig Tree and Corn plants that have traveled with us from home to home, for almost 30 years now.

I told Mother Earth about my first garden on Kingsley Street. We planted the seeds in 20' by 20' foot patch of dirt in the backyard. On the following day, the Houston skies opened up and didn't close for a month.

The seedlings never saw the sun, and I forgot again for a few years. I confessed to Mother Earth my lifelong habit of starting but never finishing projects.

I told Mother Earth of all the other gardens that I have planted since. I told her about the corn, beans, tomatoes and squash that I had abandoned. I found a place on Montclair and Nile Streets of San Diego. I'd plant once, maybe twice, and then simply forget. I confessed to Mother Earth my tendency to forget. My Wirrarika friends tell me that we live in a very distracted way. In our environment, remembering takes conscious and deliberate effort.

I can't say how long it took for me to talk about the plants, trees and the gardens I had planted. All the while I was speaking, I was very much aware of my body and the constricted space that contained it. Every once in a while, I would feel a bug crawling, or perhaps what I imagined to be a bug crawling on me. My legs itched. The grave was completely dark and the night was still. From time to time I caught a muffled sound or two that I attributed to one of my companions. But mostly my imagination and reason filled the void. I looked up and saw dark hooded images peering down at me in the grave. I saw snakes slithering in the darkness. The grave would fill with shadows for a few moments then reason would quickly inform me that the neurons in my brain must have continued firing, even in the darkness, creating images. I perceived a soft voice speaking barely audible but indistinguishable words. After a few seconds of listening, reason told me that the breath entering and exiting my nostrils created a sound that my mind converted into words. My awareness was now consistently slipping back and forth between a world explained by reason and one that continually challenged my capacity to understand.

I started talking about my human relationships, my grandparents, mother, father, brothers, sisters, children, grandchildren and close friends. One by one, I described them, telling her about my connection to each. With each relation I started acknowledging, as best I could, what it was that connected me. I found, acknowledged, and confessed a lot of resentment. I confessed appreciation, gratitude, affection, but mostly it was my resentment that kept oozing into awareness.

As I talked, images of snakes and caves kept emerging in my aware-ness. Sometimes, I allowed my attention to drop down into the caves until they vanished. I followed the serpents as they slithered in and out of the holes in the walls of my grave.

I was talking about my son Felipe and the car accident we had in 1986. We were speeding along Interstate 8 on our way to a potluck at FrogFarm when the beige Nova in front of us screeched to a stop. I veered to the right and was almost stopped when the car behind knocked our tiny 3-cylinder Sprint onto the ice plants that border the freeway. When the little red Sprint came to a stop, there was a moment of silence as every-one gathered their wits. I looked into the back seat and saw my daughter's car seat upside down in the space between the seats. I felt relieved when I heard her cry, no doubt terrified but alive. My son Felipe was terrified, but alive. Suddenly animated, he screamed out, "I love everybody, I love everybody". They say that, under stress, we speak the truth-- and that is my Son's truth. He loves everybody. I told Mother Earth about my Son and how good he makes me feel.

Having run out of my prepared speech, I was now "ad libbing." I asked Mother Earth what I should do to enjoy life more. The response was not immediate. I kept talking.

The neurons in my brain were really ramping up. I was no longer seeing dark and vague images of snakes or caves, but colorful and com-plete landscapes. The first was a field of yellow flowers. I was looking at a mound of green, covered with bright yellow flowers. The second scene was a dark, misty swamp. From here, I traveled to a mountainous region. My "reason" told me it was Tibet. I stayed here the longest, among the tall green mountains and nestled among the trees and bushes, stone struc-tures that I chose to call temples. I saw the vivid colors, and my senses could feel the bright sun that graced the flowers, feel the marsh's moist air, and the peaceful energy that enveloped the old temples. The color and the sensations completely overwhelmed my awareness.

Eventually my body grew fatigued, so I rolled over onto my left side and resigned myself to sleep. Immediately upon doing this, it occurred to me that "giving up" hurt Mother Earth. I completely understood that the

Earth "forgives" absolutely everything, but she does hurt, and I was hurting her by giving up. I rolled back unto my back, asked for forgiveness, and continued offering my awareness.

A night in total darkness and with no distraction is endless. I found myself feeling restless, but sleepy. I found myself observing my breath. As I focused on the air gently entering and leaving my body, I continued talking out loud. The words that I spoke to Mother Earth gradually assumed a life of their own. They imposed themselves and took on a rhythm. A song began welling up inside of me. It was not a spontaneous or easy flow of words and rhythm, but a repetitive process whereby each repetition became more rhythmic and coherent. After a few minutes, I was singing to the present. I let go of the past, disengaged from plans for the future, and just sang to the present. I greeted the stillness of the night, embraced the emptiness that I felt in my heart. It took a while to get the tune and all the words.

There were no places to see, nowhere to go, no fear,
No guilt, no shame to bow
My head down low
No fear in the place right here.

I sang that song a few times.

As the song faded, I became aware of a sensation an inch or two below my navel, but inside, perhaps halfway between my lower back and abdomen. At first I experienced it as an "itch", a sensation that needed scratching. Given its placement, I could not. Instead, I simply focused my attention and my breath on the spot. The sensation grew in intensity, as things do when we pay attention to them. I was not sure what to "do" with the sensation, how to interpret it, or how breathing in this situation might be useful. It simply was a sensation that grew more intense. I gently focused on my breath as it entered the spot and as it slowly escaped through my nostrils. After a few minutes, the sensation grew into an impulse to move. The thought of kicking my legs crossed my mind. I quickly realized that doing so might dislodge a slat or two and that I might find myself really buried with dirt.

Perhaps out of frustration or not being able to thrash about as I felt like doing, I began to experience the sensation as pain. Unable to contain myself, I began to rock my pelvis in an up and down motion. I continued this rhythmic, obviously sexually suggestive motion for a few moments, all the while listening to and dismissing the possible explanations, judgments, and commentary offered up by the voice of reason.

I latched on to what seemed to be the most plausible explanation. I was experiencing the pain of disconnection. I became aware that if I turned my attention inward, on the sensation and my breath, I stopped talking. So it was an effort to continue talking, but I did. Between the sensations of pain and tears, I started telling Mother Earth about the pain that I was feeling. As I did, I no longer wanted to carry or hold on to the pain that I was feeling. My voice, like the original sensation, was growing, with each breath and as my "intent" grew clearer to me. I offered the pain of separation to Mother Earth. In a loud voice, I screamed out to Mother Earth that I intended to leave my pain in the grave.

After screaming out loud, I focused on my breath for a while longer. I could see light finally filtering through breathing hole. I heard my companions rustling. Feeling finished for the night, I rolled over on my left side and slept for a few minutes. After awakening, I laid there for a few minutes more, simply listening to the muted sounds of the morning, the birds, the crackle of the fire. I left my grave when I felt ready.

In the group discussion with my companions that followed, I realized that my experience of the Earth had differed significantly from that of the Fire. Victor noted that this difference was common. Males in general seemed to have a much easier time with the Fire. I like the fire, it feels natural. Making a commitment to the Fire seemed to come much easier than surrendering to Mother Earth.

Mother Earth never spoke to me in the conventional sense. I did not hear words emanating from outside of my head. I think many of us today hold to this very narrow definition of communication, that we connect only through words. And even though in our own language, we acknowledge the "power" or "energy" of the wind, the "gravity" or "electro-mag-netic" energy of the earth, perhaps our inability to connect through words renders these as entities not connected to us. My Wirrarika friends re-mind me regularly that the Earth is always talking to us. We have simply forgotten how to listen. I know this is true. When I turned on my side to sleep, I "knew" this act hurt Mother Earth. I didn't debate it, consider or reflect. I immediately acted.

And more importantly, this truth, along with similar ones that I have learned from the *poderios*, has motivated me to continue meditation. Ac-tually it's more like praying, or simply talking to the poderios like the close friends and companions that they are, consistently every day. While the poderios no doubt support our life, ultimately through interactions with other humans that we live most of our lives. So the ritual of prayer is accompanied by a reexamination of my relationships with real people, especially my capacity to surrender, to give myself more freely. (Mother Earth's essence is to give unconditionally)!

For most of my adult life, I have privately held on to the notion that I emerged from my childhood with a hole in my heart, a sense that some-thing was missing. Through the years, I reified this vague feeling into a firm belief that my schizophrenic Mother's inability to adequately nurture and connect to me had left me a permanently damaged being, who in turn was incapable of "attaching", connecting to others. After my encoun-ter with Mother, I've accepted this notion as simply another "belief", not an irreversible "truth."

In San Diego, near the old mission dam, there is a place where the native people once ground acorns into meal. The area is called Grinding Rocks. If you ever visit, you will see massive oak trees that at first sight ap-pear to be growing out of the boulders. It's an awesome sight. In fact, these trees began as tiny acorns lodged in cracks of the boulders. They broke thorough the massive stones with the sole purpose of expressing life, of living. I know that is how life works. I know that my mother gave me absolutely everything that I needed. My own resentments disconnected me. It was not a "hole" that I felt all these years, but the weight of my own judgments and resentments that I desperately held on to. I was the one who separated. I am the one who chose to make a burden out of the life that flows though this body and through all my relationships.

I acknowledge. Better said, I *confess.*

Shamanic Initiatory Crisis

David Lukoff

In November 1981, I spent five days at The Ojai Foundation in California with Wallace Black Elk, grandson of the famous author of *Black Elk Speaks*. He had taught us traditions of the Medicine Wheel and he had guided us in the building of a sacred lodge. I participated in my first *inipi* (come back to life) ceremony in the sweat lodge that same evening.

A month later, I returned to The Ojai Foundation for the New Year's Eve celebration. Grandfather Wallace had again led a lodge ceremony in preparation for an all-night event to begin later in the evening. Wallace would lead the tipi meeting along with Marcellus Bear Heart Williams, a roadman of the Native American Church, who would drum and lead us in chants. We had consumed no food in preparation during the day of the event. This tipi meeting, unlike the traditional ceremony Bear Heart usually led, would be without peyote.

That was fine with me. Ten years before I had tried LSD for the first time. This experience had catapulted me into a two-month psychotic episode during which I believed myself to be a reincarnation of Buddha and Christ. In this altered state I had set out feverishly to write a "Holy Book" that would create a new world religion. I had weathered this episode without medication or hospitalization, but it was not an experience I wanted ever to repeat -- even though I now consider it to have been my spiritual awakening.

Early on that New Year's Eve we entered the teepee, the small group of us walking sunwise then settling in quietly. A low fire that would burn all night already gave off its glowing coals, raked into the center of the tipi and shaped into a crescent moon. The night was quite cool, and the coals gave off a warm and friendly glow.

Bear Heart began gently shaking a gourd rattle, and like many others around the circle, I began moving my head to its pleasant rhythm. He began singing prayers in Muscokgee Creek. Wallace offered Lakota prayers and I began to recognize a few words from the preceding workshop: *Wakan Tanka* (Great Spirit), *Tunkashila* (Grandfather), *Metakwe oysin* (all my relations). Grandfather Wallace had uttered those at the beginning and end of many of his teaching sessions and also during the sweat lodge ceremony.

Of course, no one was wearing a watch and I doubt my sense of time was very accurate, but the prayers and songs seemed to go on for about an hour. An abalone shell was filled with smoldering sage was passed around for us to smudge ourselves. The sage seemed especially aromatic that evening.

Then Bear Heart began drumming. He had assembled a drum by stretching an elk skin over a cast iron kettle partly filled with water. It was the familiar "one, two" heartbeat of Mother Earth, and the sound of that water drum would continue throughout the rest of the night. We did take a couple of silent biobreaks for people to stretch, drink water, and urinate. The drumming continued in my brain even during these brief breaks.

As the night rolled on, Bear Heart and Grandfather Wallace continued chants and songs. A few participants knew the songs and joined in. Most of us didn't, but at times we could add our voices, approximating the sounds if not the actual words.

After several hours, sometime in the wee hours of the morning, it started to well up within me—a sense of oneness, of being connected at a deep level. It was a feeling that I had experienced only once before, during those two months of my psychosis. It began with the feeling that I was the drumming and the drum. Then I was everyone in the tipi; I was the universe; I was everyone who had ever lived and ever WOULD live.

Then the thought occurred to me that perhaps I had been right ten years earlier. I WAS Buddha and Christ! -- OH NO!! Am I going crazy again?

I wanted to bolt out of the tipi to turn off these thoughts, but there was absolutely no way to do that without interrupting the ceremony. I took deep breaths and looked into that warm friendly fire. The drumbeat was now inside my brain as much as it was outside my body. The fire was dancing to the sound of the drumming. I told myself to focus on the fire, and that seemed to work—the drumming became friendlier.

I heard Grandfather Wallace begin another chant. I have no idea what he was singing, but it had a lilting quality and seemed quite beautiful. I focused on his singing and found myself once again appreciating the beauty of the whole scene—the fire, the tipi, the drumming, the circle of people. I had the feeling, again similar to what I had felt ten years earlier, that my whole life had been leading to this moment. I let myself enjoy it, appreciate it. My fears were transformed into a sense of well-being and gratefulness.

I have no sense of time after this point. As I slowly became aware of the approaching dawn I wondered, with some anxiety, whether these feelings of ecstasy would persist. As wonderful as they felt, I did not want to be stuck in this state of ecstatic bliss either. We arose quietly and once again walked sunwise around the circle to exit the tipi. I could tell immediately that my feet were safely grounded. We gathered to share a feast of popcorn, fruit and other light snacks that had been laid out for us by members of the Ojai Foundation community to welcome us back from our all night journey.

Later that morning, walking back to the main yurt at The Ojai Foundation, I happened to meet Grandfather Wallace on the path. I thanked him for the ceremony and managed to blurt out something about not having felt such powerful feelings since a period ten years earlier when I had been in a psychotic state. Before our conversation I had never discussed my episode with anyone except my Jungian analyst. I still felt quite embarrassed about it, and as a psychologist, I had worried that disclosing it could jeopardize my career.

To my surprise, Grandfather Wallace in turn shared that he had also experienced a series of important visions in his early 20s that had landed him in a psychiatric hospital! He had not mentioned this in any of the teachings I attended during that week. Nor did he ever refer to that experience during the next ten years when I had the opportunity to participate in other programs with him.[1]

But his sharing helped me to consider that my own experience was also a kind of shamanic initiatory crisis (Halifax, 1979) that had served as my calling to become a healer. As a psychologist, ten years later in 1991, I published an account of my journey as an initiatory experience in the magazine *Shaman's Drum*.

I also view this experience as my spiritual awakening and draw on it in my current work not only with people who are experiencing spiritual crises, but also with those recovering from psychotic disorders. I am now working with the California Institute of Mental Health to develop a spiritually sensitive approach to recovery from mental problems.

For that New Year's Eve ceremony, I thank Grandfather Wallace for reintroducing me to the world of ecstatic experience, through a ritual that allowed for controlled entry and exit from that state. I am also grateful to Grandfather Wallace for enabling me to re-interpret my two-month journey into psychosis as a shamanic experience, which contained the seeds of my future.

Halifax, J. (1979). *Shamanic voices*. New York: Dutton.

[1] An account of that period in Grandfather Wallace's life is now described in the biography *Black Elk: The Sacred Ways of a Lakota* that was subsequently co-authored with William Lyon.

Immersion, Ascetics, and the Aesthete: Cleaning the House

Elva Maxine Beach

My parents were hardcore Pentecostals, which meant-- when I was ten-- so was I. During those formative years of my life the church bombarded the congregation with films depicting the Second Coming. Every Sunday evening Pastor Wolf shouted threats of eternal doom

The month before, one of my uncles died suddenly of a heart attack. I deduced that I, too, could die at any moment. Crazy things happen. Car accidents. Drowning. Murders. If I wasn't saved and baptized soon, I would be doomed to Satan's playpen, while my loved ones enjoyed the green pastures behind pearly gates. I was desperate to stay out of hell.

I asked my Sunday school teacher what happened to children who had not yet been baptized. Her answer only baffled me more. "God loves children," she said.

Didn't God love everybody? And yet, there was this burning fire pit called Hell where He sent the unrepentant, the unprepared. Did he send kids there, too? No one would give me a straight answer; I decided to ensure that, if I died suddenly without warning, I would ascend, not descend. So I insisted on taking the baptismal plunge earlier than our church recommended.

At ten going on eleven, I stood in line waiting my turn to be immersed in holy waters. The oversized white robe the deacon gave me to cover my jean shorts and a flower power t-shirt swallowed my small frame, and I had to hold the bottom of the robe to keep it from dragging the floor. But I didn't mind. I was relieved. My days of secular life soon to be over. I was joining the ranks of the blessed, the transformed, the spiritually reborn. I was about to be baptized. Eight people had already taken their turns, and only Sister Mancha and Brother Brook were standing in front of me. I was proud to be the youngest person in a line of adults awaiting ablution.

My parents were leery about allowing me to participate in this ritual while so young; they weren't convinced that I truly understood the significance of what it was I was about to do. But after a lifetime of listening to Sunday sermons and reading Bible stories, I knew I was ready. Mom and Dad watched me from the congregation, tense and neither smiling. I waved to them, my white robe flapping like swan wings. My father motioned for me to behave, put my hand down. He frowned. I quit waving and smiling, turned to face Sister Mancha's back, and acted as serious as I could, despite my giddiness.

My parents had photo albums dedicated to the church with pictures of river baptisms from the 40s and 50s. Both of my parents were baptized in rivers, and I envied them. I was somewhat disappointed that my baptism would take place in the cement and tile pool at Calvary Temple. On the other hand, I was ecstatic that finally I was to be immersed in three-foot deep water, dunked by Pastor Wolf. I watched as he covered the noses and mouths of those before me with his hand, and submerged their entire bodies in the waters. I imagined the spiritual transformation that I would soon experience. Arising from the water, my soul would be purified, and I would grace the earth with dignity and security, knowing that my path to heaven was set.

After Sister Mancha jetted out of the waters, her perfectly primped beauty salon hair a wet mess, yelling, "Yes, Jesus, praise Jesus!", my moment came. I took the three stairs to the baptismal pool's edge, stepped down into the cool water, and felt Pastor Wolf's strong arms embrace me. He began praying as I anticipated the shock of the Holy Spirit. Pastor Wolf dunked me, once, twice, three times. Water shot up my nose. I coughed.

After the third dunk, Pastor Wolf held one of my arms in the air and shouted, "Praise be to the Lord for saving this child."

But I didn't feel saved. I felt exactly the same, only wetter. This frightened me. The baptism had not taken. I left the pool soaked, shaken, and disbelieving.

I kept my disbelief secret for as long as I could. The lack of an awakening ate at my conscious, caused me to question everything I had been taught. So when I was in junior high, I announced to my parents that I would no longer be attending services at Calvary Temple. "It's important to me to find my own path to God," I said. They looked at me as though I spoke a foreign language. Yet, as distressed as they were about my announcement, they let me be. They didn't try to coerce or persuade me to change my mind. They didn't ground me or punish me like I had expected. Dad said, "Babydoll, I have faith in you. Your mom and I will pray for you."

I was lucky. My parents had been primed for religious rebellion by my brother, who was 13 years my senior. Ken had already experimented with drugs, hitchhiked across the country, delved in glam rock, punk rock, and was an off-and-on hippie. In 1979, Ken returned home to live with us and dry out from his overindulgence in the counterculture. He had turned vegetarian, started running marathons, and taught my Ozark-raised, uneducated parents about healthy diets, meditation, and alternatives to the concept of God.

My parents, although neither of them finished high school, were not stupid. They watched the world change around them. They lived through a depression, World War II, the Korean War, and Vietnam. They witnessed and approved of the civil rights movement and women's liberation. They were disgusted by Nixon, the Watergate scandal, and the chipping away at unions and workers' rights. They were barely aware of sub-cultures like the beats and hippies, but they knew and accepted that times were a'changin'. So they allowed me to stop going to church.

One value they refused to let go was the concept that cleanliness equals righteousness. Hippies were okay, they admitted, but they needed to bathe more often. My father lived by the axiom, "Cleanliness is next to Godliness." So as a youngster I equated the Pentecostal immersion baptisms with the first step to this holy cleanliness. My disappointment with my own baptism caused me to question not only the validity of my church but also the metaphoric ritual of a baptismal cleaning. I became a pragmatist. Perhaps, cleaning ourselves, absolving ourselves of sin, meant doing something more practical.

When my brother explained fasting to me, it all made sense. I reasoned that when Christ commanded that his disciples be baptized, perhaps he meant internally baptized. Fasting rids the body of toxins, and toxins could be equated to sins. The translations that I had been taught of holy texts could very well be wrong. Christ was known for his healing powers, and if fasting helps our bodies heal, than maybe through fasting I could become closer to God, could be healed of my "sins." And if Dad was right, and our bodies are our temples, then yes, fasting is a true form of baptism.

In my attempt to be "clean" I fasted for almost two days. I hated it. I felt dizzy, hungry, discombobulated. And my brother was not a patient mentor. My first fast was ruined after about 45 hours because I used toothpaste when brushing my teeth. "Toothpaste is the same as food," my brother roared. "It has sugar in it! You can't brush your teeth when you're fasting!"

Ken should have been thrilled that his 14-year-old baby sister, who up until a couple of years ago was a die-hard Christian, would even consider fasting. Had he looked around, he would have realized the teasing and bullying I endured from the neighborhood kids for attempting something as nutty as not eating. It was 1979 after all, and people in working-class neighborhoods like ours did not fast. People in my neighborhood ate meat with every meal, attended church on Sundays, and prayed like they were choking.

The whole world was tipped upside down, and my spiritual development seemed to follow the same backward and inside out pattern as the world in which I lived. In spite of the radical changes I was making in my lifestyle and my belief system, I maintained a yearning to merge with and honor God with my actions, and cleanliness of some sort was a path to unity with that greater force. Also, I admired my brother, adored the new ideas he brought home to me (meditation, vegetarianism, yoga, Zen Buddhism). And fasting seemed to be the epitome of the "cleanliness" thrust of most religions.

I tried fasting again, the second time lasting for three days. The third time, I lasted a day and a half. The fourth time, I gave up on the first day. It was difficult suffering, my belly grumbling, my energy zapped, my normally enthusiastic perspective turning dark with hunger, teenage angst, and a burning realization that this ascetic life was not for me, any more than being a practicing Pentecostal.

After my baptism experience, I felt cursed. Through my high school years I felt guilty, not being able to go the distance with a fast. Then around the age of 19, I had an epiphany. My brother's path was not my own. Food is one of God's gifts. Our enjoyment of his gifts is one way to honor him. I should relish and explore food, not deny it. I'm closer to God when I'm enjoying the pleasures of life. I'm not an ascetic; I am an aesthete!

I love long, hot baths. Taking baths creates the perfect space to quiet my chattering monkey mind. So, for a few years into my young adulthood, I used my bath time as my private ritualized baptism for God. I kept my hair, nails, and skin immaculate. But (Perhaps because my sensuous baths required no suffering), my daily bathing ritual did not produce the transformative results I was longing for. This schism between the ascetic and the aesthete haunted me for years. I was lost. Taking pleasure in the creator's gifts should not be at odds with honoring the creator through some type of ritual with water and the spirit.

Over time, I have recognized the holy in the mundane, and have come to understand that each small action we take creates beauty or causes ugliness. Our choice. I have also discovered it is in simple tasks that we often find answers to complex questions. No doubt my father influenced me in this sphere, as well. When I was growing up, Dad often pointed out our neighbor's broken windows, uncut and littered lawns, unpainted houses and said, "Just because you're poor, doesn't mean you can't have dignity. These people should take more pride in their homes." *House-proud* is the term.

I keep a clean house. First-time visitors in my home often comment on how immaculate it is. I usually smile and thank them for the compliment and leave it at that. I don't explain why my place is pristine. I have found my own form of holy baptism in the act of cleaning house.

I'll admit cleaning my body and home is also a response to my anxiety, my tensions, my feelings of being out of control. Cleaning calms me, and in cleaning not only do I find a quiet mental place, but also I feel transformed along with my floors and walls and counters and sinks. It is miraculous to me that something as benign as water and soap can change the face of disrepair. Cleaning my home (or my friends' homes, or my office, or anything) solves my ascetic versus aesthete dilemma. While I am scrubbing, say a bathtub from gray to white, I feel like one of those young monks who enter the monastery to find his primary task is to scrub floors, or like a young soldier in boot camp who ends up spending hours toiling away with a toothbrush cleaning the bunkhouse. The labor and discipline needed to clean something properly satisfies the ascetic urge.

As far as sating the aesthete – look at any clean dwelling and there you will find beauty.

Most of us, except the most slovenly, have some sort of cleaning ritual, whether washing the dishes or intricate cleaning rituals. So mundane, so pointless-- whatever you're cleaning will just get dirty again, right? We may fail to see that by dousing our surroundings with water and soap, we are baptizing our lives and honoring our gods.

When I wash the dishes, dust the corners of doors, scrub a bathtub or sink, make my bed, wash and fold clothes, vacuum, scoop out the cat box, wipe the counters of my house, I discover peace and lose myself in an otherworldly meditation. When I am engrossed in this daily activity, I am transformed just as much as the things that I am cleaning. The disappearing grime and resulting glean fuels my hope that all forms of darkness can be washed away, given enough elbow grease. The fundamentalist baptism (being dunked in three feet of water by a Pentecostal pastor) and the more disciplined cleansing (starving myself in order to rid my body of toxins) do not compare to the holy joy I feel when performing my favorite cleansing ritual. On the floor, on my hands and knees, supplicant, washing away the dirt my chaotic life tracks in.

Moving Beyond Chaos

Issadora Saeteng

Bright innocent shining eyes
The child's face did glow

Her radiance, joy, happiness and love
All of this and more did show

Daddy's girl, mommy's princess
The only world she knew
Came down and tumbled on earth
As a meteor drops from the moon

Assault occurred on dreary days
Death seemed so sure
Pain so deep,
She couldn't quite feel
Frozen into place

Trapped, alone,
Confused, terrified…
Life as she knew it,
now gone.
Drained away
like blood from a slain animal
heaped in forgotten soil

Would she live?
Would she die?
Did any of it really matter?
What? Why?
What happened?
The world may never know…
It so happens in this case
The child was rescued
Returned back to her safe home
But then set in the aftermath of pain
The pain so deep, it numbs…

Flashbacks, memories
Convergence of time,
Dissociated spaces
Reality undefined.
Night after night
long fear-filled times
She lay there avoiding sleep
To calm the nightmares,
Trying to make them go away.

This pattern of action
Wasn't working
Sleep had to come
Nightmares overtake
No peace could be found…

How to organize chaos?
Inner chaos felt so strong
Yet untouchable from the outside
Chaos living, breathing inside her
Sapping her life away

So in what we call rituals
She discovered
Methods to alleviate this deep pain

Long hours of silent prayer
Based in reality of the day...
Preparing her bed
Soft cuddly animals
A reminder that she is safe
A reminder that she will be fine
A reminder that God is here
A reminder to continue faith

Holding her bear, she said a prayer
She thought about dreams she wanted to have
She willed her brain to come up with images
Of Penguins on a slide
Around and up and around and up
They went and went and went
Soon enough, she fell asleep
And went with them too
Around and up..
Around and up
Safe and close
Safe and secure

Books by day
Fantasy, adventure, fiction, non fiction
It didn't really matter
The point was experiencing
The point was safe
The point was God is here
The point was faith

And soon in time
The flashbacks went away
The nightmares dropped off the scene
Dissociation never really quit
Survival was key.

Trauma hides many secrets
Memories hide away
the body never forgets
But ritual helps take the concern away.

The girl grew up into me
I survived
I'm here
A reminder that I'm safe
A reminder that God is here
A reminder that I'm strong

Unraveling the Knots of Negativity and Soul Pain with Simple Rituals

Joseph Rubano

I WOULD LIKE TO OFFER THREE PIECES. THE FIRST TWO ARE EXAMPLES OF spontaneous and semi-planned rituals for healing wounds arising from relationships -- the first is a spontaneous ritual that arose for my own healing; the second came out of my role as counselor, partly planned and partly spontaneous. The third is a morning ritual that I have been doing for a couple of years. Relatively new to my conscious attention, it may be of importance to many people today: a ritual of connectedness to the place where one lives.

About four or five years ago, someone very close to me acted toward me in a way that hurt and angered me. The exact situation is not import-ant. What is important is what arose in me as a response. I was hurting, and knew that I needed to do something to process the hurt. I walked around on my front deck feeling the pain and anger, picturing the person. As I was stewing, a spontaneous image arose. Probably because ritual and ceremony have been important in my life for over 20 years, I was able to recognize the fleeting image as an invitation to ritual.

The image was, *breaking a beer bottle*. Strange image, but I immediately recognized the healing it offered. Beer is the beverage of choice for my dear friend who stimulated me so. I went into the recycling bin by the garage and picked out an empty bottle that I was pretty sure he had emptied. I walked around with the beer bottle in my hand and opened myself to what to do next. Beach rocks are arranged in many places on the deck, and I began collecting some. I knew that I would need four stones for the four directions. I drew a circle in the deck to contain the ritual that was being formed.

I place the four stones in the four directions, acknowledging them one by one. I place the beer bottle on the stones. I kneel within the circle in front of the stones and bottle. I feel my hurt and anger. I pick up another stone, a bigger one, and allow the feelings to grow. I raise the larger stone above my head, and with a sound coming deep from my belly I shatter the bottle.

In an unusual calm and silence I sat with the shattered glass around me. I felt relief. I felt cleansed. Then with a relaxed humility and gratitude I slowly picked up the pieces of broken glass. First the bigger pieces with my fingers-- realizing that this slow picking up of the pieces on my knees was part of the ritual; it felt sacred and important. I swept up the smaller pieces and placed all the pieces in a bag. I ceremoniously picked up the stones and returned them to where they had been. The stones were not the same stones that I had picked up-- they had been changed along with me. They were now ritual objects.

For hours I felt free and open. Eventually my mind kicked back in, and a familiar negativity came back. But remembering the ritual, a smile came, and the negativity faded away. This happened several times, but each time the negativity had less power. A few days later I was able to talk with my friend. An understanding was spoken and heard, and it was done. A new story was created for the life and love between us.

This ritual unraveled a deep knot inside me. It had the three elements that give ritual the power to transform negativity: having a clear intention, being connected to feeling, and getting the body involved. Intention, feeling, and active doing.

***

One of the things I do is counsel people. I had been counseling a man and a woman who had been in a love relationship for several years, but now it had ended. They wanted to remain friends, but they had been in this transitional space for months, churning up all kinds of unhappiness and blame and resentment. They could not make a clean break, and they could not be with each other in a good way. I had the idea to do a ceremony to help dissolve the invisible ties between them, to help them acknowledge the ending of one relationship and the beginning of another. Healing from separation is possible when faced directly and honestly, with dignity and beauty.

They were both willing. I had them think about what they wanted in their new relationship, what their relationship had been for them, what the gifts of it. I asked them to think about what they most valued in the other and to find something that signified the relationship-- their hopes and dreams, the gifts, the pain. I told them that we would use a fire to burn whatever they wanted to release, to let die, to be transformed by the fire.

When we met I lit a candle and burned sage. I acknowledged that we were here to serve the highest good, and asked for help to honor what needed to be honored and to release what needed to be released. We went out to the chiminea in the back yard, where I had the wood already set and waiting. I lit a match, and we sat watching the fire grow. I spoke of why we were here and invited them to speak. They each spoke, looking at each other, looking into the fire. Tears and laughter. They spoke prayers to each other, beautiful and moving. They each placed what they had written and spoken into the fire. They stood facing each other. Then spontaneously I walked over to the juniper bush and broke off two sprigs. Handed one sprig to each of them and invited them to bless each other with the juniper sprig, touching different body parts as I spoke: "*Bless the eyes that you may see clearly and find beauty wherever you go, that you may see the right way for you to go; bless the ears that you may hear the sounds of life around you, that you may be open to hear what is difficult to hear, that healing music can fill your soul; bless the mouth that you learn to speak only what brings beauty and healing, what helps life and love to sprout around you, learn to speak the truth even when it is difficult to speak, may you feel free to sing the joy that is in your heart ...*

And we went on touching and speaking to the heart, the lungs, the back, the shoulders, the elbows, the wrists, the hands, the fingers, the belly, the hips, the legs . . . the knees, ankles, feet, to the toes. We acknowledged the gift of being human and wished blessings upon blessings. After the final blessing to each other, we laughed. They looked into each other's eyes and placed the sprigs into the fire.

Each drank from two glasses of water I'd set out. We thanked each other and ended.

The dance between the two has not ended. Now about eight months later they are not in a sexual relationship, but their friendship is deepening. They both report how important the ceremony, to establish a common ground and to remind of their intention to continue their relationship in a new and healthy way. The ritual, witnessed by a third person, helped to free up old knotted places and give power to their love and their desire to create harmony and friendship. I think the ritual gained power and magic in that we were outside with the wind and sky, with fire and water, standing on the earth. Experienced with their whole being and all the elements present, we also used the power of speech and touch as healing and blessing.

*****

I mentioned a ritual of connectedness to the place where one lives. I have been meditating every morning for over 35 years, so that is not new. What is new is the connecting with the land and beings of the land right outside my house-- my place on this earth and my place connected to the heavens. I feel this conscious connecting is important nowadays when so many of us feel rootless. I am learning how to be rooted; it is a relief.

After I wake up, get out of bed, roll around a bit to work out the morning stiffness, I go outside. I greet the day by speaking my greeting. It goes something like this:

I am Joseph. It is a new day. I am the one who walks upon this earth, step by step upon this earth where I live. I walk in the morning on this ground that supports me, this earth that nourishes me. I give thanks for the firmness beneath my feet, to the sprouting green, to the gophers who live beneath, to the worms and dead leaves. I am the one who speaks and who sees and hears and who speaks what I see. I turn to face the sun and feel its warmth. I turn and close my eyes and see the orange glow behind closed eyelids. I give thanks for you sun that rises each day that brings light and warmth, that gives rise again to the colors of the trees and grass and flowers and fruit. That lets the sky be blue and me to see. I give thanks for the clouds and the birds. For the beauty of their flight, for the beauty of their song. Thank you for the bird song and the movement of the leaves in the wind, for the bright orange of the oranges and their juicy roundness. I say good morning orange trees, and lemon tree, and grapefruit tree. I say good morning old and twist-ed plum tree and budding peach. I say thank you hummingbird that perches each morning on the top branch of the plum or orange tree, that disappears in a blink of the eye, that flashes green and red and makes me smile. Thank you for always being there.

I say it is a good day and I am alive today. And I say this day may I bring beauty, may I bring life, may my heart be full. May I remember how the stars are my home, that this earth is where I stand. That this earth is a star and I am a star and bring light with each footstep I take. May I walk in beauty this day.

And then sometimes I sing or chant or simply breathe and expand my field to include all sounds and movements and forms around. Then with eyes closed I sit breathing, feeling into the space of the heart until I am ready to enter into the busyness of the day.

This daily ritual takes 20 to 60 minutes, depending on how much time I have and how long it takes to allow the spaciousness of the heart to become a felt reality. This simple beginning of the day gives meaning to my daily life. It reminds that I set the anchor for my life in place. I look forward each morning to feel the breezes to touch the earth to look up into the sky to speak. This speaking almost feels like a necessary responsibility-- that the trees and sky and sun and moon and birds need my speaking as much as I need to speak.

Thank you for this opportunity to share this with you. I am Joseph Rubano -- I am the one who speaks and is grateful. *Aho!*

The Healing Power of Music: An Anecdote on Ritual and Release

KEN GILL

RITUALS ARE FOUND IN EVERY ASPECT OF OUR LIVES. FROM THE MORNING rising to the sports field, workplace, church and all points in between, we all engage, consciously or unconsciously in ritualistic behavior. This anecdote on the healing power of ritual revolves around music, performance and audience.

First, as with any ritual, the preparation. We had several nights booked in Sedona, Arizona, with a nine- piece show band I had toured with in the '80's. It was going to be fun as well as a serious amount of work. I had to chart out all the songs, burn CD's of them and put together and mail off a binder for each player. This all had to be done well in advance so each member had time to prepare. Along with all that of course was learning and rehearsing all the material myself.

I had to go through my equipment from stem to stern and get it road-ready. I would be driving out from San Diego for two days of rehearsal prior to the gigs. Having a very full-time job, a loving wife and twin six-year-old boys (all of whom were coming later to join me in Arizona), all this extra work, while exciting, pushed me to the point where I was exhausted. Not long before I had to leave for Sedona, my back went into spasm, and I was in bad shape for the task ahead.

Ever since I was young, the instruments and accessories that go with them have been very special to me. Acquiring good quality instruments, amplifiers and effects devices was not only costly. It had taken years to find and accumulate the reliable, top quality equipment needed to play professionally at a high level. I gain satisfaction and comfort just dealing with the tools of my trade. The packing, setting up and taking down of "the stuff" is a precise ritual that I have performed ever since I started playing professionally at age 15, over forty years ago. So I left on my trip in high spirits but physically very restricted in what I could do without lots of pain. Lifting and loading the gear and the more than eight-hour drive did nothing to help me mend.

Arriving in Sedona, where I had lived several times and played so many gigs, was wonderful. The beauty of the red rock country only added to my pleasure at being back with my mates. Meeting with the members, and the entourage, all like brothers and sisters to me, with all the miles traveled and all the joys and drama shared, was exhilarating. During the two days of rehearsal, the familiar ritual of set-up and practice was helping me to temporarily forget how painful it was to do basic things, like bend at the waist.

The high energy of performance was of course absent in rehearsal, with all the starts, stops and corrections being made as we went through the song list, working on remembering the nuances and parts played so many years before. When performance time arrived, nervous anticipation was at its peak. The sudden release of it when the first powerful notes erupted from our speakers made it like . . . no time had passed. The intervening years were swept away and we were laying it down hard and heavy and rockin' the house. When the performance is rolling, the crucial element of an audience lifts you up like a wave. By the third set, which came all too soon, I was enjoying the effects of the rising energy in the room. My pain, while not gone, was at least "sitting out" until the break between sets.

I am normally very physically animated on stage. Not only does this increase the entertainment quotient, it's just plain impossible to stand like a stick when the groove is deep and insistent. In the third set was a special number, which grew over the years from an improv based on a rock hit from the '60's, into an epic psychedelic event. Years before, we had played for ten straight days, (four of those double shifts), in Prescott over the Fourth of July. During this period, Prescott attracts large numbers of bikers. Their hogs line the streets for blocks. One night, a large, bearded biker approached me on stage and asked, "Do you know Purple Haze"? I had played Purple Haze, the hit song by Jimi Hendrix, years before in high school. I told him I used to know it. To which he replied, "You know Purple Haze." Not having the size or inclination to disagree with him, we launched into a rendition of the tune pulled partly from memory and partly from thin air. Jimi Hendrix gave himself totally to his performance, using not only his gifts as a musician, but also acrobatics and tricks to please the crowd. I attempted to put a similar life into our admittedly hacked version. The patrons, most of whom were large, bearded, and under the influence appreciated my efforts and responded loudly. Even the bouncer, a taciturn, stern faced, large bearded biker himself, started treating me nicer.

Over the years of touring, that improvised piece grew and morphed until it was fifteen or more minutes long and included several other Hendrix tunes as well as everything from sea shanty's and Motown hits thrown in for fun. It also became a physically demanding performance, during which, in order to be true to the sprit of the music, I had to keep escalating the intensity and showmanship every time we did it. Some nights you may be tired or not in a flamboyant mood, and you hide that when you play. For this piece, I had to reach down deep and truly let the beast out of the bag! This night, at this point in the evening, six of our members left the stage, leaving me, Dave the bass player, and Stanley the drummer to carry the next 15 or more minutes.

Even though the ritual leading up to this or any performance is much the same, once I count it off, it is different every time. As the electronic thunder exploded from my amplifier, I found myself transported, feeling the power of the music and the energy of the audience flowing through and wrapping around me. I sang, played, leapt and cavorted about the stage. At one point I was on my knees in front of my amplifier coaxing soaring waves of feedback from the equipment. I lay back, knees on the stage and my back on the floor, caressing the humming instrument in my hands and-- as Jimi said in a song-- "Lord knows, I felt no pain".

After the song ended I felt light, elated, potent. Once the evening ended, the afterglow of performance lasted through the takedown and the after-party at our hotel. The only thing missing was the near debilitating back pain, stiffness and muscle spasms that had plagued me for the past week.

The complex ritual of preparation, rehearsal and performance had culminated in an energetic interchange with my band mates, the audience and myself. The energy that passed through had taken us all to a place where there was no pain, only the incandescent wonder of the moment.

For a link to to access his music, email *Ken@san.rr.com*.

UNLEASHED

LESLIE ZIEGENHORN

YOU MAY REMEMBER TOTO'S MISCHIEF IN *THE WIZARD OF OZ*. DIVERTING Dorothy from her plan, Toto often added unwelcome chaos to the mix, forcing the entourage on a scenic route at the most inconvenient times. Yet it was the dog – an extension of Dorothy's own instincts and animal knowing – who deepened her journey by calling attention to otherwise invisible importants. Ultimately, it was Toto who blazed the trail to the Wizard, and with one tug revealed the disillusioning truth behind the curtain. For Dorothy, it was a matter of opening to it, meeting it, and realizing the necessary losses inherent in the inevitable wake of change. Revelations may be waiting where we least expect them, and where we least want to look.

It is Dorothy's connection with Toto and her willingness to allow his spontaneity to lead her to awe that parallels my experience of "ritual." My ritual has not involved a regimented discipline, but daily walks inspired by the eager press of dogs to explore the world beyond cornered walls. While other kids were being socialized with Barbie dolls, Big Wheels, and "playing house," each day I was living out my own version of Oz, exploring Kansas farmlands and woods with a variety of dogs. Some were our family pets, and others joined the pack as they saw us trekking to the majestic kingdom the neighbors called "the weeds." Years later, my Kansas weeds yielded to Michigan wild lands to the California canyons where I now live.

Any place where the wild divine weaves its magic (which may be everywhere), and any *creatura* who encourages engagement with that (which may be anything), are sufficient ingredients for transport. As the experience seduces me to open to what is present, I begin to commune with mystery. Ordinary time, space, and consciousness become sacred. Dorothy's path to discovery was paved in yellow bricks. Mine was dirt, creek, and meadow. Both of us followed Toto.

My current Toto is my dog Tex, and Oz waits just beyond my front door. Our daily adventures begin in the suburbs, which, as safaris with Tex reveal, can hold many delights. Yards spotted with newsworthy markings from local dogs require her close attention. Anything resembling a plastic container warrants a detour, and the garage that housed a Pop-Tart years ago remains on the roster. For the two-legged voyeur, the neighborhood's landscaped gardens can be delightful. Burying my face in the silky lushness of a domestic rose, for that moment I relish knowing nothing beyond "It's so *pretty* to be alive!" But the pruned roses, like the preened lawns throughout hardcore suburbia, create a sort of false Eden – a place where signs of death are often quickly cut and whisked into airtight containers for the next trash day. The gardeners and landscapers, however, get the full story, from seed to fruit to decay to seed. Just so, hearts break and families dissolve via slow death, infidelities, divorce. Unless the Wizard's curtain is pulled back to reveal the brief presence of a U-Haul filled with a vanishing portion of the home's furniture, you might actually believe you are enjoying someone else's paradise.

Just beyond civilization's tidy lawns, where the pavement yields to dirt, is a trailhead. Liberated with a click of the leash, Tex and I prefer immersion in perfectly unkempt wilderness. Nature, the great Nataraja, serves as a constant calibrator. Each moment birthing, sustaining, dying, pausing, rebirthing. Surrender to this splendid play of life - far grander than our personal dramas - composts personal grief, glory, doubts, lust, naiveté, shadow and light. One may sense the Infinite before, behind, above, below, you. There is still plenty of "pretty," but unlike the domesticated yards, death is always an undeniable backdrop, centerpiece, or next scene. Something divine is unleashed in the grandeur of Nature feasting on itself.

Of course there are many places, grand and tiny, where this sacred feast occurs. Its magic can be woven almost anywhere. In the depths of the ocean, on webs in the windowsill, across mountain vistas, under fingernails, in tropical jungles, inside a table vase, within autumnal forests, between cracks in sidewalks, deep inside caves, amid vast deserts and on the bottom of your shoe. For over a decade the Tecolote Canyon in Southern California has been a particularly special teaching, playing, grieving and sniffing grounds for Tex and me. Tecolote is a Native American word for Owl, and on some lucky twilight fallings, we have heard them there. Even more rarely, we catch a shadowy glimpse. *Swoosh!*

While daily treks have birthed countless stories over the years, one in particular comes to mind when I consider the revelatory potential of the ritual dog walk. Not far from the Tecolote trailhead, there is a little clearing in the oaks that occasionally surprises me with a new pile of rocks atop freshly turned earth. An Animal Graveyard. These piles stand as a marker of some child's grief, an initiation to impermanence and the other side of love. I am saddened, but Tex is curious. Then I'm curious, too. The size of the rock pylon invites me to wonder what beloved pet lies beneath. Some piles are hamster-sized, or maybe a goldfish loved as big as a hamster. A parakeet perhaps? A midsized pile could be a guinea pig or an iguana. At times there is no guessing. Fixed atop some gravesites may be a photograph or Crayola drawing of a cat or some other dearly departed. Sometimes taped to a makeshift tombstone, these pictures are often sealed tight in plastic baggies. But alas, eventually the color fades to indiscernible hues, and beads of moisture invade the sealed bag, acting as foot soldiers of inevitable decay.

During one hike, her keen nose on high alert, Tex's course to the graveyard was so determined that it nudged my morning sluggishness toward a mild frisky. When we neared the rock piles, her sniffing grew more fervent, and my curiosity quickened. She led me to a freshly dug hole, dirt splayed haphazardly around its periphery. It was a big hole. Bigger than a hamster, for sure. Tex followed her nose down a flattened path of ground foliage that created a trail leading out of the hole into the riparian scrub.

With a peculiar seriousness, she examined a swath of ice plant. Her ribcage bellowed as she unraveled the mystery, as if the entire sordid story was revealing itself through smell. Eyes narrowing and ears back, Tex lifted her head and paused as if considering a retreat from the scene. She tentatively resumed sniffing, sniffing, sniffing. I resumed looking, looking, looking. Looking into the hole and along the flattened dragway toward the creek, I struggled to coalesce the clues into a discernible story.

"Oh. What's this?" A scruffy hairy something. Tentatively, I looked sideways out of one eye, both horrified and fascinated to see whatever was there. "Hmm…" Just a longish wiry thing, coarse black hairs mixed with grey. Brows furrowed, I inspected it for signs of its former incarnation… no paws or ears, but a nubby remnant of vertebrae. Suddenly my curiosity gave way to disgust. "Oh God, it's a *dog's* tail!"

Upon that unsettling recognition, the stench of death filled my awareness. I grimaced, but as I started to look away, something on the rotting tail caught my attention. Something…moving? I held my breath. I drew my face closer. There, atop the very tail that once wagged joy at reunions and sagged when scolded, was a maggot. As my focus narrowed onto its white formless body, the maggot pulled one of its tips upward as if checking me out, too.

At that moment of mutual curiosity, a shaft of morning sun splayed over the canyon wall and illuminated the maggot. It lifted itself up further, and, no joke, puffed out its chest, glowing in apparent triumph over my horror and disgust. There it was, emanating the robust energy that peaks at the prime of life. Vibrant and radiant. I could not deny its beauty. I could not deny its conveying…that Nature *will* feast on itself. Like the dog and its tail, even the Maggot, the Glorious Maggot, will return to the earth. Never again to live in that particular form. Eventually the last trace, including any memory of it, will fade into ephemera, its existence composted into the yet unknown. At that moment, the archetypal lesson of impermanence imprinted deeply within me, even deeper than the many unwelcome reminders that had come before. There was a shift. I felt simple. Vast. Connected.

The encounter with the maggot was a portal. It bridged a more intimate dialogue with the chaotically precise installation of color, form, textures, tastes, and smells of the Earthly Divine. My daily ritual deepened as I began to consciously step out of my voracious mind and become more soulfully present to the rich panorama before me, communing not through language or concepts, but through direct experience of what is. A tiny, formless carnivore of decay illuminated the way. Within the ordinary lies the seed of the extraordinary, and magic is birthed from the mundane.

The maggot's gift is in every moment, if only I fall awake to its offering: The glowing backlit plumage of a red-tailed hawk gliding effortlessly, making otherwise invisible forces gorgeous to behold. A fragrant fennel bush buzzing with bees; I close my eyes and put my face to it, my restless mood transformed by the vibration. The iridescent crimson flash of a hummingbird's throat. Tiny flowers with perfectly aligned petals, pinstriped and intricately decorated. Lustrous moss carpeting a rock. Bizarre pods and spiky things that appear just in time for Halloween. The ghostly presence of a blue heron, silently staring into me with one sharp eye. A mushroom springing from an other's refuse, now standing like a proud flag declaring, "Something pooped here!" A smeary glimpse darting into the hole I had passed by many times without ever noticing. The translucent sepia husk of a locust, now somewhere else sporting another body. A swift ribbon of shakti traced by a vanishing snake. The erotic darkness lining the eyes of a coyote, mystically materializing from the thicket then vanishing. Mating insects excitedly pairing on a specific day due to some particular alignment of elements, assuring that the life-force expands itself through form as masculine and feminine find each other in the magnificent chaos of it all. This morning it was a spider village splayed across the canyon grounds, the previously secret webs made visible only for a moment when sunlight illuminated the dew at just the right angle. Countless little miracles reveal themselves if one is present. The Maggot, of course, is among them.

Lately I try to soak up the wonder of it all without glossing over my own sadness on these daily ventures. The challenge lies in my growing capacity to experience awe and sorrow simultaneously. The teacher, again, is Toto. The shorter lifespan of most other animals allows us to observe the entire arc of life. The inherent lesson of impermanence is a hard one to bear, but a necessary honor to witness nonetheless.

Once a surrogate mother to Tex, a tiny pup I found in the New Mexico desert, I am now a midwife to death as I watch her 15-year-old body return to the earth. Tex's decline is a stark reminder that my body and all the glory around me is following suit. Her once graceful and effortless stride is now cumbersome as her front legs move like stiff but determined sticks hauling her atrophied hindquarters behind. Occasionally a leg gives out. She is surprised by the collapse, but makes a trusting recovery as I lift her boney frame back on the trail. At these moments, I recall her younger years, when she boundlessly kangarooed through the thickets to rustle out critters, circuitously covering at least eight times the distance of any one of my linear miles. Our current meandering now requires a slow patience that I would frustratingly resist were it demanded by anything less than love. With her eyesight clouded by cataracts, Tex uses her nose as a divining rod that leads us to ever more obscure patches of off-trail earth. I now have no choice but to witness different little miracles we would have never known under other circumstances.

What's this? Tex's muzzle nudges the dirt. Among a delicate scattering of bleached white bones – a tiny perfect femur.

RIP Tex - Run in Peace
Good Life, Good Death
August 30th 2010

****

"...No matter where we are, the shadow that trots behind us is definitely four-footed" Clarissa Pinkola Estes

"For years, copying other people, I tried to know myself. From within, I couldn't decide what to do. Unable to see, I heard my name being called. Then I walked outside."
Rumi

"...you will gain the great freedom of giving yourself to life...you will be able to squander yourself into life...healthily as nature squanders herself. Then, and only then, will you know the beauty of living."
Eva Pierrakos

Personal Experiences with Ritual

RICHARD SEIGLE

A Ritual with Starman

I WAS AT A PICNIC ON THE REZ AT MY DINÉ ("THE PEOPLE" AS THE NAVAJO want to be called) teacher Eugene's home. His mentor Starman was there. He was looking at me. Eugene walked over and said that Starman said I had a lot of *hocho* or negativity to clear. He explained to me that most people need one or two rituals for their problems, and then they are clear until they pick up more *hocho*. In the counseling or medical field you pick up negativity that can build and build until you get sick or burnout or make a change.

We drove down to his ceremonial Hogan. I sat on the ground in front of a small fire, and Starman started smudging me. When he was ready, he stood in front of me and Eugene supported me from the back. Then Starman proceeded to put his forehead to mine and push as hard as he could. He then did the same thing to my chest and abdomen. I was supposed to give up all my *hocho* and negativity in a shamanistic way. Because I was scared, I felt that I had not surrendered completely. When he was done, Starman walked over to a shopping bag and spit out this black stuff.

Several months later Starman would do this again, and then I surrendered completely. After I cleared my body and mind through prayer and rituals, I was able to feel and avoid negative energy. I could feel *hocho*, then try to protect and clear myself as much as possible. A good way to do this was by smudging, or by participating in a sweat lodge ritual (the oldest ritual in this hemisphere).

A Ritual with Eugene

When Eugene came to visit San Diego for the first time in 1988, I wanted to show him some of the beautiful areas we have here. When I took him to the top of Palomar Mountain, he lit a cigarette and we stood in silence. After he was done, he explained that he was praying with native tobacco. In his way, the smoke carried the prayers up to Great Spirit. It meant to me that ritual could be in any place in any moment. When we were in La Jolla, I explained that the Native people used to live there. He looked at me and said, "I know, we used to live everywhere." This was very sad and humbling.

Learning about Negative Energy or Hocho

My first critical/crucial lesson came when I showed Eugene the seclusion rooms at the hospital. He asked me how they prepared the rooms for the next patient. I said, "They mop the floor and make the bed." He said to come outside. Eugene stated that patients in seclusion were troubled by negative energy or they were more susceptible to it. If that energy was not cleared or cleansed from the room, the next patient would be exposed to it so on. This was the first time I heard about negative energy and a dark side to things. Maybe I was a bit naïve, but my training had not given me this information (we spent one hour on Jung in three years). Something inside me clicked and I understood why I had been run down for months.

When Eugene did his workshop on healing rituals that weekend, I got in touch with my soul and my purpose that had been dormant for many, many years. I steered a new and spiritual path for myself. I added ritual to my life, initially, to offset negativity from patients in my practice. My ritual was smudging myself before I came in the house. When I was comfortable bringing sage into my office, I smudged before I left the office. I started feeling better, and early morning patients would comment on the freshness of the office. Eugene also recommended some kind of shield or protection over my heart.

Sometimes, when you put your intention and commitment to attention, things happen that begin to satisfy what you were asking for (or get worse to show you what you need). Sometimes by the time the ritual comes, your requests have already been answered -- and you can be thankful for this in the ritual. In ritual, you can go back and clear out things that you never could remember or clear. It is not uncommon to start crying, become fearful, or have emotions of happiness and love. The medicine man called it the roto-rooter of the mind. When you get on a spiritual path, there are things you can no longer hide. You start to have more unconscious or repressed memories move towards consciousness. There are things you can no longer avoid. Why keep running around in circles while we are racing head-long to our death?

Helping People with Ritual

I first helped a person with ritual when I treated a nurse with panic attacks. I was trying to help Liz (not her real name), who in the past had tried many types of therapy. About six weeks into treatment, she was still stressed by career decisions and wanting to get pregnant.

With permission from the therapist and the patient, I asked about the family tree to see if there was anything negative that could be affecting her now, subconsciously or unconsciously. It is common for people to have an ambivalent or negative relationship with their parents or stepparents. In this case it was Liz's stepfather.

Her preparation for the ritual was extensive. She had already taken up yoga at my suggestion and really liked it. I asked her to do a complete family tree and we talked about problems in it. We focused on other negative events in her life that still bothered her. Finally, I asked her to write down what she wanted or needed in life in the way of affirmations.

We set a time for her friends to come and support her, and Liz told her story. Some of her friends had not known all her trials, and Liz revealed one important detail that I had not known about. There was great negativity to clear in this instance and we were able to do that.

When I saw Liz a month later, she was feeling better, even happy, and hadn't had any more panic attacks. Liz showed me a picture of her mother in a white wedding dress, which meant a lot in terms of clearing negativity. Liz called me a few months later to tell me she was pregnant. One could say that Liz could not be a mother until the situations around her mother could be accepted.

Can someone have an easier time getting pregnant after a ritual? In the Bible, Jacob's wife cannot get pregnant until she makes a covenant with God. Could her belief make a difference? Of course! A feeling of safety and healing can decrease anxiety and give the person peace and acceptance of how things are. They can let go, so to speak, because the ritual proposes a state of *hozho* (balance, harmony, beauty and wholeness). Imagine how the brain and body changes the hormones and neurotransmitters to balance the body biochemically. Balance in body, mind and spirit and allow a pregnancy to move forward, where it couldn't before.

Over the next few years, I worked with many patients who asked for a ritual because they wanted something in addition to their traditional treatment. I was doing a prayer ritual for a couple with a few of their friends. I spoke about mother earth and father sky and how the Diné believe that we are cradled between them. After I was done, the woman to my left spoke about growing up with alcoholic parents. Talking or thinking about her father and mother would upset her, so she avoided that pain. She said that now she would think that she was being cradled between mother earth and father sky, her new parents. Insights like these relieve anxiety and discomfort, not with medicine or therapy but almost instantaneously with intense "symbolic psychotherapy" (Topper, 1987).

Spontaneous Remission

Before a healing workshop I received a call a few days from Brenda, who said she could not come. I pressed her for the reason and was told that her mammogram showed a mass and she needed a biopsy/excision. She wanted to stay home and focus on her problem and not be around people. Gently, I reminded her that this was a healing experiential workshop it was meant to help with one's problems. I was saying this because some people think these rituals are of some interest and don't really help or they are coming because they are curious. Brenda came after all and received a blessing but was private in the group and only a few of us knew that what she was asking for. Brenda had also used visualizations until the time of her biopsy. After focusing on the mass for days, she saw it finally burst apart and then she could no longer focus on anything in that area.

When she came in for the surgery, she asked for another mammogram. The doctor said that would waste time and they were ready to operate now. She said she would not sign the consent until she had a mammogram. They did 12 mammograms and could not find anything. You would think that the surgeon would want to know how this happened but instead he came into her room and threw down her paperwork, saying, "I don't know what happened but you had some kind of spontaneous remission."

RITUALS FOR UNRESOLVED GRIEF

There is another very important aspect fulfilled by rituals that we don't think about in western medicine, which focuses on the "identified" patient. Diné believe that, since we are all connected our family and loved ones need to be brought into balance as well. Dr. Robert Nemiroff of UCSD said that unresolved grief could account for 80% of the people that go into therapy. How many people say, I wish I had told my mom how much I loved her before she died. It applies to a father, sister, wife or friend. Having a healing ritual with others allows them to do, say and feel what they think about this person they might lose or want to get better. If there is a loss with unresolved grief, then in a ritual you can say what needs to be said and can let that person go.

For millenniums, rituals have been used to heal. A ritual can happen in a moment in any space or may last days. The goal of Navajo healing is to bring the person into Hozho (balance completeness, beauty), close to what Jung wrote in a letter about his work helping the person achieve the numinous (pertaining to the spiritual), a connection with and balance of their spiritual life.

A ritual may answer one's prayers or not. A negative result or a lingering issue may happen because that is how the universe is, positive and negative, health or illness, life or death. If you have a "successful" ritual, then the outcome doesn't matter. The outcome will be as it should be, accessing the numinous.

An example of this was a ritual for a man in Shiprock who was in the hospital.[1] He was brought into the sacred space on a stretcher with an intravenous line. We prayed all night for the man, even though he had to leave after a few hours and return to the hospital. The man died, but he knew that the ritual had done everything for him and it was his time to go. In other words, in the divine order of things, the gods have been summoned and responded, as it should be. The ritual made sure that the man wasn't dying from negativity. A ritual can empower someone and make them strong and move into acceptance in the stages of loss. How should we prepare for death if "God wills it?"

Stages in Healing Rituals

Martin Topper, an anthropologist who had also studied psychology at UCSD, found that the Dine' ceremonies were quite comprehensive. If put into western psychological terms they consist of purification, confession, therapeutic alliance, transference, suggestion, intense symbolic psychotherapy, extinction of anxiety and the reconstitution of ego defenses.

The first stage in healing rituals is clearing a sacred space, purification. A ritual should take place in a sacred or precious place, but any space that can be made sacred. The negativity needs to be cleared. Rituals can be for happy and grateful and celebratory times. At this point, all negativity should be dealt with and removed. Then comes the personal story of what is wrong or why they need a ritual. This is the confession. The story of how we came to be at this point is revealed. Total exposure is preferred to clear all the negativity.

The next component is the healing. This is difficult to describe because it varies. One component of the ritual might be passing a talking stick from person to person so they have a chance to ask for what they want or need. It is hard for some to speak or pray in public and ask for what you need. Sometimes it takes a long time to face your demons and get out what needs to come out so the healing can come in.

The final stage is the blessing. This is for all participants, the community, all the creatures and elements and the earth and on and on. After this is done, the sacred space must be honored and anything from it carefully handled or removed.

I like two quotes that describe rituals more generally:

"Rituals surround us and offer opportunities to make meaning from the familiar and the mysterious at the same time.... They engage us with their unique combination of habit and intrigue" (Imber-Black & Roberts, 1992, p. 3).

"The rituals in our lives contribute to our changing sense of ourselves over time, while also connecting us to the generations who came before us.... They can provide an opening into ways of being and beliefs that both affirm our own and are totally different from our own" (Imber-Black & Roberts, 1992, pp. 305–306).

Ritual can help because the mind is the most powerful healing tool we have, and love is the most potent power for healing. Unfortunately, the mind can also make us ill or put us into a living nightmare of confusion and contradiction.

Using ritual with proper preparation can make life-long changes and promote healing or acceptance of one's sacredness and connection to the divine.

References

Imber-Black, Evan and Roberts, Janine (1992). *Rituals for our times: Celebrating, healing, and changing our lives and our relationships.* New York: HarperPerennial.

Topper, Martin D. The traditional Navajo medicine man: Therapist, counselor, and community leader. *Psychoanalytic Anthropology 10:3* (1987): 217-49.

RITUAL AND THE ART OF RELATIONSHIP MAINTENANCE

AIN AND AMY ROOST

DECK/FIRE TIME

AIN: FROM THE VERY BEGINNING OF OUR RELATIONSHIP AND WITHOUT ini-tially realizing it, we established several relationship rituals that subsequent-ly evolved into sacred relationship time. The first of these is deck time. This basically involves sitting out on our deck, usually with our legs up, taking in the view. We have been fortunate enough to have excellent views from our various decks during the time we've known each other, most recently of the ocean. Having a distant vista is a helpful component of deck time. It facili-tates the long view, a big perspective with a sense of open space. Things are not crammed into it. Things open up and patterns are easier to see.

We sit and look out, most often a sunset, and then the night sky, an even more distant vista. There may be a glass of wine, or Pelegrino, per-haps some cheese and crackers, and sometimes, in our British moments a spot of tea. We gaze out, let our thoughts wander, and things just bubble up. It's essentially free association. We share, we talk about our day, we catch up on each other's news, we make plans. Sometimes we deal with issues that need to be addressed. Sometimes we blue-sky, our term for expansive thinking about the future--projects, plans, dreams.

We both feel a freedom during deck time. There is no pressure to say or do anything. We're just hanging out together, sitting and enjoying the view. Whatever constrictions that have occurred since the last deck time are allowed to breathe and open up. It reminds me of my introduction to meditation. It was 1970 and the Beatles brought Maharishi Mahesh Yogi and Transcendental Meditation to the Western world. In my initial orientation my teacher Lynn Napper described the process. Our individualized mantra would function like sonar directed into the depths of the ocean. It would sound out our depths and bring our issues to the surface, thereby increasing the possibilities for understanding and productively processing them. The "not doing" of deck time is similar. Whatever is under the surface is allowed to bubble up into our awareness. Our dialogue, often about things that we ourselves may not have been fully aware of, allows greater self and mutual understanding, processing, and often loving resolution.

Amy: I'm going out on a limb to say that not enough couples make space in their lives for deck time. I certainly didn't in my first marriage. With the competing demands of career and raising children, taking the time to sit down and check in with my husband seemed like a luxury. In those days my mother used to offer to watch our children so my husband and I could go out to dinner. More often than not, I'd thank her but say we couldn't afford to go to dinner. She'd always respond, "You can't afford not to."

The same could be said of deck time. Ain and I feed our relationship much needed nutrients every time we carve out space in our busy lives to tend to each other and our relationship. Not carving out this space translates into sweeping dirt under the rug in hopes that it will go away.

On a personal level, part of the reason deck time works so well for me is that I feel supported, emboldened, almost anonymous, with a vista upon which to focus, especially when discussing difficult issues. The larger perspective takes it beyond just the two of us; the universe is a witness and a party to the dialogue. Any silences during deck time are easy, and when I do speak, my words are chosen more mindfully because it feels like there's a line on the horizon connecting us to one another and to the larger wisdom of the universe.

Ain: A variation on deck time is fire time. A fireplace, a fire pit, a camp fire or even candles can create the same feeling of space. Space seems to be an essential dynamic. Space allows us to step out of the often hectic, agenda-driven, goal-oriented schedule of our everyday lives into a separate reality.

If you have a fire in a relatively dark space it's almost impossible not to find yourself gazing into it. It's hypnotic. Something on a very primal level draws us to fire. As a magnet for our attention, fire was kind of the original TV set in the cave. However, fire as opposed to TV allows our attention the freedom to wander anywhere and everywhere. Fire is fluid and moves continuously, in a flowing graceful dance, that just like snowflakes never repeats itself. It's endlessly fascinating. And the "not doing" of this fascination elicits much the same kind of sounding out of our depths as a distant horizon or the night sky. Free association and sharing of whatever comes up will inevitably ensue.

Fire has another aspect to it that I think goes even deeper into our primal roots than appreciation of the visual fluidity. We are actually encountering the source of our existence, interacting with our origin in the big bang and the resulting galaxies and stars, one of which is our life-giving/sustaining sun. As children of the stars we are literally made from fire. That fire in front of us is a part of the sun, as Thom Hartmann described it: it's ancient sunlight. The fossil fuels that we burn in a fire are stored up energy from the sun. The sun nurtured the plant life on earth, which in the form of wood, oil, etc. we burn, thereby releasing the energy of the sun into light and warmth. The sun, stars and fire all have the same element in common, which in some primal way connects us to each other.

Both of these dynamics contribute to the free-form thoughtfulness that takes us away from the everyday mundane chatter of "monkey-mind" and connects us to ourselves, each other, and our "big sky mind"-- in sacred time.

Amy: When Ain and I sit by the fire--generally holding hands or entwined in some way--I have warmth; I have shelter; I have love. In short, I have security. Is it any wonder that I can open up to him and express my deepest fears, desires, wishes, thoughts?

Cuddling & Snuggling Time (AKA The Stations of the Cross)

"You do not have to walk on your knees
for a hundred miles through the desert, repenting.
You only have to let the soft animal of your body
love what it loves."

-- Mary Oliver

Amy: This is the second ritual from the beginning of our relationship. Truly there was some greater underlying intelligence of which we were not initially aware. We believe it was our mutual attunement to the soft animals of our bodies that we allowed to have their way with us. Later on our heads caught up with their wisdom.

Each morning when our alarm chimes, Ain rolls over on his back--if he's not already there--and extends his right arm. I scooch over from my side of the bed, and, laying on my left side, place my head on his right shoulder and drape my right leg over his hips. As our bodies meet, it's not uncommon for one or both of us to let out a sigh as we melt into the home of each other's embrace...aaaahh. This is *Station One* of three in our morning cuddling ritual.

Depending on who's more awake, one of us will begin, slowly at first, to move our hand across the skin of the other. I'll rub my hand across his chest or down his thigh. He might play with my hair or massage my ear lobe. We might ask each other "how'd you sleep?", or I might share a dream I had, depending on how awake I am.

Station Two involves Ain rolling onto his right side to face me. My breasts meet up with his bare chest, and I keep my right leg draped over his hips. I might rub or scratch his back, he mine. We both experience a phantom satisfaction from touching the other in places and in ways that we ourselves love to be touched. For instance, I know how good it feels to have my back rubbed and scratched, and thus can get almost the same satisfaction scratching his back as I do when he scratches mine. This no doubt has something to do with mirror neurons. A mirror neuron is a neuron that fires both when an animal acts and when the animal observes the same action performed by another. Thus, the neuron "mirrors" the behavior of the other, as though the observer him/herself were acting. More simply put, it's kind of a monkey do, monkey feel process. Our touch is not only pleasing the other, but has a self-soothing effect as well. Eventually we move on to other parts of our bodies that get less attention, like armpits, wrists, elbows, feet or even webbings between the fingers.

We might be talking in full sentences by the time *Station Three* rolls around. We'll compare schedules and perhaps talk about upcoming plans as I roll over to my right side and we "spoon" with each other. He will caress my breasts, my stomach, my neck, my ears, and I'll reach back with my left hand and massage his scalp and we'll feel the warmth of our soft animals going "mmmmmhmmm...".

In its entirety, The Stations of the Cross ritual lasts maybe 15 minutes, and we set our alarm clock early to reserve time for this important ritual. The Stations of the Cross is more of an intimacy ritual than a sexual one; the morning ritual is more about sustenance than anything. It is one of the ways we feed our relationship and keep it healthy. My husband has artfully described it as follows:

OXYTOCIN JUNKIES HAIKU

CUDDLING AND SNUGGLING
ESSENTIAL PART OF OUR DIETS
OFTEN NEGLECTED

On the rare days when we skip cuddling due to our schedules, both of us feel "off", even skin-hungry, much in the same way you might feel if you regularly ate breakfast and had to skip it one morning.

While it may seem basic to cuddle with your partner, with busy lives over time there is a tendency for important things like this to drop out. By ritualizing our cuddling we've made certain it's not overlooked. It's what we do when we wake up, like opening our eyes, stretching and getting out of bed. It's that simple.

Ain: Yes, we're definitely hooked. I think this ritual became known as "The Stations of the Cross" from my initial position--on my back with both arms spread--and the subsequent ritualized nature of the sequence. The loving nature of the mutual holding and touching has a soothing devotional feeling that seeks to make the other person feel good and simultaneously creates the same feeling for ourselves. It's a variation of social grooming among animals, a health-maintaining, trust-building, bonding activity that's beneficial on multiple fronts. It's a gentle caring, soothing process that wordlessly tells us that we are home in each other's arms and that all is well. We are loved and held, and anything that needs to be healed begins to heal.

FEEDING TIME

Ain: This ritual has evolved over time, primarily during the making of salad for our dinner. A wonderful salad is almost always the first part of our dinner. Sometimes it is substantial enough to be the whole dinner. We usually have a mixture of lettuces and herbs, to which we will add an assortment of nuts--selecting from a menu of pistachios, sunflower seeds, candied walnuts or pecans, slivered almonds--and vegetables. Whoever is making the salad will avail him/herself of the chef's prerogative--sampling and sharing tidbits during the preparation. Sliced avocado and tomato along with pickled asparagus or hearts of palm are almost always part of the salad, and provide tasty little morsels to have and share with each other.

Once we actually sit down to eat the finished salad, which is always a delectable treat, we relish the finished product. However, the tasting and sharing during the preparation has already been a wonderful part of the event and has become its own ritual.

Amy: Part of it I'm sure has to do with the somewhat naughty feeling of eating some food before it's actually table-ready. Many of us when we were little kids had the experience of sneaking some part of a meal before the preparation was finished. Given that mothers often objected to this practice, it involved getting away with something, and sometimes getting scolded if we got caught. So there is something vaguely illicit that has to be part of its charm. Or sometimes mom would recognize the exquisite delight of a preview tidbit and grant us the privilege. As adults, who can make the decision for ourselves, it still feels like a sort of exceptional abundance.

Ain: Offering these little morsels to each other sometimes literally involves placing them in each other's mouths, kind of like mother birds feeding their young. There's something kind of tender and nurturing and loving about it, on both ends of the process, the giving and the receiving. And usually there is a warm feeling and a little smile that goes with it that has a sense of connectedness, caring and being cared for.

Amy: One the greatest satisfactions of motherhood (and now grandmotherhood) was feeding my children when they were too young to feed themselves--watching them open their mouths as they saw the spoon approach, eager for the offering to their expectant lips. I'm sure mine was an instinctual feeling since mothers are hardwired to nourish their young. What I feel when I feed Ain is very much the same: "Open up, person that I love, and receive some of what sustains life."

Ain: And then there's the sensuousness of the taste and texture of the offering. The nutty taste and the creamy texture of a slice of avocado in your mouth, all by its sweet, simple, complex self before it joins the party with the other ingredients. The sensuousness of opening your mouth to the offering from your lover's hand, your lover opening her mouth to what's in your hand, trusting in the goodness of it, and each other. Being nourished and nurtured.

Amy: Maybe it's the Italian in me, but I can also think of few things more sensual than food. Truth be told, the seductress aspect of feeding Ain is most appealing. I'm a Goddess offering my God some peeled grapes. Or naughty Kim Basinger offering Mickey Rourke some strawberries and chocolate. As rituals go, feeding each other has many alluring dimensions to it.

The Healing Game

The process of regularly sharing these rituals nurtures and helps heal our relationship on a continuous basis, both proactively and retrospectively. The "healing game" is an ongoing process in life. There doesn't have to be any huge dramatic injury for healing to be necessary. There are rifts and tears, dings and scratches in all of our daily lives, from numerous sources, big and small. Cleansing and ongoing healing is an essential part of healthy maintenance, of ourselves, each other, and our relationship. Clean as you go works as well in relationships as it does in the kitchen.

These evolving relationship rituals have served us well over the years. Our relationship somehow keeps getting stronger, and we believe that these practices are an important part of that. They allow us to transcend what we previously understood to be the boundaries of relationship. Transcending, we observe, integrate and transcend again, in a recursive process that allows these two "strange attractors" to create meaningful, satisfying patterns out of the chaos of our daily lives. As we step out of our insular selves and attune to each other we greet the light within each of us, and through that we gratefully resonate with the energy flowing through the universe.

A Personal Journey of Meaning, Love, and Ritual

Susan Murati

Albania was an unknown to most of the world: a dark, secret place whose borders were closed for 50 years by the communist regime. When democracy overthrew the regime in 1992, I was one of several trainers hired for an American-sponsored school for ex-political prisoners and their families in the capital city of Tirana.

Fortunately, my Peace Corps service in Ghana in the mid-70s prepared me for Albania's poverty, lack of central heating, sporadic periods of running water and electricity, and the absence of most conveniences Americans take for granted. My co-workers and I became nighttime scavengers looking for canned soup or rare rolls of toilet paper in one or two stores in the city that carried these items. We made a joke of it, but life was very tough for the Albanians, whose average wage was about 15 dollars a month.

As I settled into the routine of Albanian life, and learned some of the language, several Albanian families invited me for visits or an occasional meal. These visits are rituals that demonstrate the importance of human connection, of formalized respect, the love of hospitality, and the importance of relationship. A visit is a vehicle for communication, for transmitting news, for arranging business and marital engagements, and other social and cultural matters. Throughout the years of communism, when the majority of families lived in poverty without telephones, television, computers, automobiles, or other forms of communication and transportation, the visit was a means of social survival. The dialogue was the lifeblood of the culture. What appeared to be gossip from my perspective was the fabric of trust, involvement, decision-making, and serious life concerns.

During a visit, drinks, sweets, and coffee are offered in a slow and relaxing prescribed order. The host or hostess leads the conversation with a series of formal phrases and responses, asking about the health of family members, work, and other matters of personal interest and courtesy. The give-and-take of the questions and responses is respectful and comforting. Albanians place a sacred honor on the act of hospitality and of being or having a guest. When you are my guest, I am responsible for your life and safety. No harm may come to you.

Even today, the host or hostess may place pillows behind a guest's back so that he or she may rest more comfortably. S/he may place sheepskin rugs beneath the feet, as shoes are most always removed at the door (If you haven't rested your bare feet upon a thick sheepskin rug, you haven't lived). In olden days the hostess washed overnight visitor's feet. On one occasion when I stayed at the home of an Albanian village family, I was "tucked in" at night.

One day I visited a woman, Semiha Aliaj, who would later introduce me to her brother Asllan. He was a well-known chemist from Tirana, whose parents hailed from Kosovo. Just one year after setting foot on Albanian soil, through the ritual of visiting—and the ubiquitous Albanian obsession with matchmaking--I accomplished a life-long goal: to marry a wonderful man.

After the second year of my contract, Asllan left Albania to become an American immigrant, and later an American citizen. We were to live, work, and study in several U.S. states, returning twice to Albania for extended visits.

But I get ahead of myself. It was more than a social introduction that made this match. For the feast day of Saint Anthony, my students asked me to accompany them to an annual ritual at a mountaintop shrine at Lac, a small town in the north. Here Albanians walk up the mountain to a sacred place dedicated to Saint Anthony, doing so under the cover of night during the communist regime. They prayed for miracles; they prayed for cures; they prayed for hopeless cases. Here was the place of miracles, and my students knew I needed one.

We boarded a train in Tirana, and soon arrived at the station in Lac. My five students advised me to buy the prescribed number of candles to pray for all of my relatives. We were to sleep on the mountain all night, along with about 5,000 other hopeful and faithful pilgrims. Perhaps more than half of them were Muslim or Orthodox faiths; there were no distinctions at this shrine. All Albanians knew of the power of God at Lac, and everyone needed miracles.

Before I left Tirana, I knew that I would ask God and Saint Anthony to help me find a good husband. Over 40 years old, I had been searching with no luck. We walked up the mountain quietly and reverently. Many of the devout walked barefoot up the rocky dirt trail, for extra indulgences or perhaps for deeper meaning known only to them. There was an air of excitement and fun, as well as solemnity. At the top of the mountain some young men carried a statue of Saint Anthony. The faithful touched or kissed the statue and placed offerings in a box. We milled around like ants on the top of that mountain, ants who were happy to have arrived at exactly the right place at the right time.

My students (all Muslim women between the ages of 20 and 25) began searching for a place to bed down for the night. They had brought food, and we had bottles of water for drinking and washing, so important in Muslim culture. We spread out some blankets. As darkness fell, we lit small fires—soon there were hundreds of small fires along the mountainside, and in the neighboring hills. We later lit our candles, one for every family member or intention, and we prayed silently. For the first time in my life, I put it clearly and directly-- and even somewhat assertively-- to God, to help me. Lac was the place for this. I wanted the right man, a good man, a man chosen by God.

Soon after praying, I heard light strains of music from the top of the mountain, tunes of African American spirituals, such as "Swing Low, Sweet Chariot"! I often wondered how those sweet melodies made it to the top of a mountain in Albania. I took comfort in the sound, late at night, as I prayed with 5,000 Albanians for all our hopes and dreams to be heard by God on the mountain, under the stars, with candles and small fires glowing all around us. We slept a little, or perhaps just rested and felt the power of a multitude of people gathered for prayer.

It was a community ritual: cathartic, public, unashamed, joyous, authentic. Ritual is like that. Ritual involves belief and trust. Ritual is passed down through the generations, natural because it has been repeated and valued, become real through practice, through "stepping out in faith." in this mountaintop ritual the faith of Muslim women in a Roman Catholic saint was as fervent as the Catholics and Orthodox. I was healed and renewed by my participation.

In the early morning we said goodbye to St. Anthony, gathered our things, and quietly walked down the mountain. We took a path lined with wildflowers. At the bottom of the mountain we found water flowing near some rocks, where we washed our faces and hands. My students chattered happily, satisfied with the night. We took the slow train back to Tirana.

Ten days later, Semiha Aliaj introduced me to her brother Asllan. It just so happened that a month before the same feast day of Saint Anthony, Asllan's brother Ramadan had insisted that Asllan make the journey up the same mountain to the same shrine, to ask God for help in finding a wife. And so we met and were married. On my wedding day I had perfect inner peace and knowledge that God had answered my prayer, and had sent me Asllan out of love and caring and His almighty and sacred grace. As I walked down the aisle of my church on Cape Cod, Massachusetts, I felt the blessing of God, and I knew it was right. We had no big wedding reception or bells or whistles, but I had God's stamp of approval.

In our 12 years of marriage, besides being an ideal husband, Asllan became my guide to the Albanian culture, with its wonderful rituals. Living in his home, we received hundreds of visitors and paid visits to hundreds of family, friends, and neighbors. Neighbors became friends partly because Albanians are great talkers and storytellers—like my Irish ancestors. We attended weddings and pinched the cheeks of many children, always saying the right things to ward off the "evil eye."

Over the years I heard quite a bit about death and the rituals of death, because Asllan's mother was called upon to help prepare bodies of close friends and neighbors for burial. Asllan's father had driven a truck to transport mourners to the cemetery. On one trip to Kosovo in 2002, the legends of the dead became apparent to me, after the war and the forced march of Kosovar refugees into Albania. As we visited Asllan's cousins, we heard stories of death in the accounts of the war from every family. Each one had its unique trauma, memories, and legends.

In a 6-month visit to Albania in 2001-02, my husband's brother Ramadan (Dani) became ill and died in the hospital in Tirana. I received the call from Semiha. "Be careful!" she screamed, in a panic. "Ramadan is dead." She was warning me to take care of Asllan so that nothing would happen to him. We had just visited his brother in the hospital the day before. Dani's health had not been good. Like most Albanians, he had smoked cigarettes for years. He had been under stress.

Over the next 12 hours (and the next several days, and weeks) Dani's death created an explosion of activity. The family, friends, and neighbors re-enacted ritual practices based upon of generations of death and death ceremonies. They cleared rooms on Ramadan's side of the family home, preparing for the arrival of the body. Couches and chairs seemed to fly through the windows and doors. Caring friends and neighbors cleaned and rearranged. They purchased coffee and cookies to be served to the mourners, who would be coming steadily to the home for 40 days. Ramadan's three grown children were summoned from Germany.

Dani's body arrived in a casket and was placed in the living room. The mourning began. Muzejen and family and friends began to speak, wail, and cry to him, asking questions: "Why did you die so young, and leave me here alone? My spirit, my dear one, my husband, why did you go? You were my good husband--- my spirit! My love, why did you go? Why did you leave your wife here alone? We were here, speaking together, we were eating bread and drinking coffee! Come back! Why did you go so fast, so young, so soon? Ramadan, we miss you! I miss you!"

"Oh, Dani, why did you leave us here, your sisters? You were just here with us, staying with us, and now you are gone! Why did you leave Muzejen? You were driving, you were going to Germany to see your son and your daughters, Oh Ramadan, Why did you go? Why did you leave your daughter, why did you leave Gentiana, and your son Beni, and your daughter Bana? Come back to us! Come back and drink coffee with us! Come back here, oh, Dani, come back! You died so young, so early, so soon!! You left so quickly!!"

As cousins and groups of neighbors and acquaintances came, the waves of grief poured out. The mourning grew, and grew, and grew, came to crescendos, quieted down. I was able to join in the mourning as I gathered the strength to express myself: "Why did you leave your brother Asllan, you were two brothers, and now he is alone!" I wanted to grieve and mourn, but I had never expressed grief aloud. In fact, throughout my Irish American life, I had hardly expressed grief at all. I had felt sad and empty. I had cried. But never before had I mourned. Never before had I faced death so directly. Never before had I smelled death or tasted it.

I was never one to "fake it," but in the middle of the outpouring, I had to find my voice, to participate. I needed to do it because I was suffering and needed to give voice to my anguish. Mourning affirmed my life and my relationship to the deceased and his family—my family. The more I said, the more I wanted to say, and the more in touch with his death I became. This was right, good. The ritual of mourning in the Albanian style healed me; it made me whole.

Each day I prepared lunch for the mourners at my husband's home. I shopped for meat and fruit and vegetables. I prepared soups and salads, sometimes with Muzejen's friends or my husband's relatives. Each morning I threw buckets of water down the stairs of my husband's home, and down the driveway, sweeping the area clean with a hand broom in the Albanian fashion. The flowers were beginning to bloom, and there was life and light outside at the beginning of every new day. The cool water cleaned the air as well as the cement steps and patio. It helped me to feel connected to the ritual and the family. It prepared the area for the full expression of grief. The cleaning of the area, the opening wide of the gates, the gathering of the family at our home for lunch, the assembling of the mourners for wake-keeping----- all of these activities and more were the Albanian rituals and customs of death.

On a rainy dreary day the Muslim cleric or "hogj" performed the ritual songs and prayers associated with the burial. Riding in a car in a cortege behind Ramadan's casket, we spoke with a woman who had recently lost her child. In the rain, grief poured out, in a cultural playing out of emotion. Others' stories of death were reactivated, Recognition of death was everywhere. Our suffering was channeled into mourning and remembering.

Like marriage, death had eluded me for over 40 years. When my grandparents and other relatives and friends had died, I was always far away. Death now caught up with me in Albania. As a child, I never heard talk of death. I heard nothing about Ireland or the conditions there or the details about the decisions leading to emigration. There were no legends— only a vague impression of suffering. I had to "fill in the blanks." Indeed, I was afraid to ask. Perhaps the Irish cultural past had been too painful.

In 1995 Asllan was diagnosed with cardiomyopathy—an enlarged heart. He had a big heart in every meaning of the word. As time progressed, his heart condition finally led to his sudden death on the morning of May 12, 2005, just three years after his brother's death. We were far from Albania and his relatives. I was alone and in shock. One of my brothers and an Albanian couple and my Lebanese neighbor helped me with the arrangements, but there was no support system as in Tirana. My church became my center of ritual, as we planned the wake, funeral, and burial. God had made my marriage possible, and God was seeing to the end of it.

Some of his relatives arrived on the second day. We postponed the wake and funeral until we brought two of his sisters from Albania. I had prepared the funeral home for the needs and customs of the mourners, and I tried to make arrangements for some of the outpouring of emotion that I knew the family would need to express, even on their first hours on American soil. I stood at his feet, as his sisters entered the room. What can I say? I will never forget that moment, as I tried to pave the way for them to do the mourning they needed to do. *Llani, your sisters are here! Your sisters!* We mourned as best we could in that funeral home, but . . .

My personal mourning for Asllan was delayed. His relatives returned to New York on the day of his funeral, and his sisters Albania shortly thereafter. My Irish coping style kicked in, perhaps due to anger that I cannot describe. Feelings of resentment and silent anguish replaced my true mourning until the duties were done and the relatives were gone. Shock and numbness remained after hysteria left. I could not cry out in public as I had in Albania. Perhaps my grief was too great, or it was too private. My comfort came through prayer and crying that poured out over the days, weeks, and months. I took comfort in my work. Even if alone in my grief, strangers and co-workers and my neighbor comforted me.

I remembered Asllan telling me about how he once threw himself on his mother's grave after her death, alone at the cemetery, in an effort to console himself. And so I did likewise, alone, throwing myself on his grave, trying to draw comfort by imitating him, but my shame made me rise up quickly to avoid being seen. I smoked cigarettes at the graveside, placing one lit for him on his stone, in the Albanian tradition. I lit candles and remembered not to say "goodbye" as I left. I wore black for 40 days, and I wore no makeup or lipstick for months, also in the Albanian tradition. These rituals and observances helped me to pay respect to his memory.

We gathered as a family in a restaurant in New York a few days after the funeral, when his family hosted an elegant lunch. Here we missed Asllan and paid him respect, together in our black clothes and our grief. And 40 days after his death, his family and friends gathered again on Cape Cod in the Moslem tradition, and we again remembered him at the grave and placed flowers and sang and cried, lit the candles and placed the symbolic lit cigarette on his grave. One year after his death I traveled to Albania to host a lunch with his Albanian family and friends as a memorial tribute. For his 2-year anniversary we gathered again.

I had to deliver Asllan's eulogy when I was still in shock, and it was quickly scripted, not adequate or right. My legend of Asllan is developing and forming from his stories of 50 years in Albania and his journey throughout America. I knew him in both worlds. He was "… the best chemist in Albania." He had inventions, he won awards. He often said, "I want to honor myself, my family, and my country." He had his American legend, too. He was a passionate, patriotic man who loved America with all his heart. He often said, "I was born in America." He loved people—all kinds of people. He embraced it all.

As I look back, my eulogy to Asllan was merely a brief brushstroke. I want to do it over again. But looking back, I know that I was helped by Saint Anthony and blessed by God.

THE PRESENCE OF MOTHER EARTH IN RITUAL

SHARON G. MIJARES

SINCE ANCIENT TIMES RITUALS WERE USED TO EXPRESS OUR RELATIONSHIP with heaven and with earth. Ancient people recognized the relevance of ritual for personal, cultural and environmental healing and connectedness. For the last three thousand years, many of our rituals (for example, the Mass in Catholic services) have ignored Mother Earth in holy rites. In this chapter I share how my creation of a personal ritual space in order to form a deeper connection with Mother Earth-- one that would later contribute to my work with women's healing groups.

During 1989 through 1991, I was a student in Matthew Fox's Institute of Culture and Creation Spirituality (ICCS) in Oakland, CA. Students lived together in dormitories, and many had traveled from nations around the world to learn methods for self-discovery and cultural transformation. Almost every course in the program provided training for participating in and leading ritual and experiential growth processes. The majority of our rituals honored the feminine and her presence as Mother Earth.

I experienced the strongest evidence of the power of Mother Earth on my birthday October 17, 1989 -- one month after enrolling in the ICCS program. I was in my dorm room resting after class. Shortly after 5:00

p.m., there was a knock on the door. My roommate got up from her own bed in response. A nun from Brazil was standing at the doorway with a balloon to wish me *Happy Birthday*. At that moment the 1989 Santa Clara County/Oakland earthquake began. My roommate from Los Angeles, and I from San Diego, knew this was a strong quake. We looked at one another, our eyes expressing a *knowing* glance. As we all rushed for the doorway on the fourth floor of the dormitory building, a print of a Shaman woman with her eagle spirit came crashing to the floor, minor evidence of the power of this earthquake. As we would soon learn of the nearby devastation, the Oakland Bay Bridge had collapsed -- during the evening work hour rush. Many students gathered in a large garden on campus as Starhawk, a Wiccan teacher, led a ritual to the Earth Goddess. The ritual gathering provided a space to affirm our respect for Her power, while providing a healing space for many frightened students. I realized that my first task the next day would be to bring peace to myself, and to then provide healing for traumatized students.

Whereas that earthquake had wrought destruction, I was soon to experience another earthquake – one that did no harm. This second earthquake occurred three or four months later. I had been given an assignment in creative writing class. We were asked to go outside, connect with nature, and then write from the perspective of a plant (or a piece of wood or rock, etc). I had found it difficult. Then the thought came to me that I wanted to write as though I was Mother Earth Herself.

Typically I walked up a nearby hill just before sunrise—usually with two or three friends. As the first step of my ritual to the Mother, the next morning I went for a sunrise walk in a redwood forest. The goal was to feel connection to earth as I walked through the forest, and to then return to the dorm to follow through with the writing course assignment. I first meditated to quiet my mind – to ready myself for learning from the archetypal Earth Mother. I "ruled" that the words had to come through me directly, without pausing or to "think them out." With pen in my hand I recorded the following message,

You walk upon my paths and acknowledge my beauty
But you do not know my power--

*The power that can push forth mountain peaks
and open valleys for oceans to fill.*

Gaia, our Mother Earth, seemed to be speaking through me as I recorded Her message. I paused, awaiting the next phrase, but the message did not continue in words. Instead, the earth began to tremble. She was manifesting Her power as it shook the earth. Later I would learn the epicenter of a small earthquake was at this spot. The words had spoken of earth's beauty and power, and the earthquake, synchronistically validated this declaration.

Whereas this ritual had been planned to create a space for creative writing, it turned out that something much larger was taking place. Think of this! The feminine (and nature) are often portrayed as beautiful (a term used for both women and nature), but her "power" is rarely acknowledged. The power of nature-- to move mountains, to shift continental plates as oceans fill the vast spaces between them, and to produce new life-- is immense. Does a woman truly recognize this force within her? Do we even know how feminine power would differ from masculine power? The earth's capacity to shift the ground beneath us comes from a deep source.

How many women affirm this inherently spiritual, earthy power? This affirmation of feminine power has the potential to heal untold numbers of women living their lives without manifesting their potential. Due to the dominating influence of patriarchal religions, the majority of the earth's female population has little, if any, awareness of the Goddess tradition. For this reason, feminist psychology and spirituality always note the role of historical and political elements in shaping women's limited identities. But in the last few decades-- due to work in the fields of historical, archaeological and anthropological research-- women have learned that pre-patriarchal history tells a very different story. Rites and mythologies from Goddess-worshipping civilizations affirmed the feminine. Archeologists and cultural anthropologists have brought to light this hidden and timely knowledge, and rituals help to evoke and to ground ancient webs of feminine connectedness.

In my women's groups I always begin our rituals with that gifted message from Mother Earth.   We begin by evoking the elements of fire, earth, air and water, along with the powers from above (celestial forces) and below (unconscious shadow forces), and then repeat *"You walk upon my paths and acknowledge my beauty—but you do not know my power— the power that can push forth mountain peaks and open valleys for oceans to fill."* We add *"Blessed Be Our Mother Earth"* as a way of affirming that beauty and power.

This structure underlies whatever theme which seeks to enable both personal and communal development.   The rituals themselves may address issues of aging (maiden, mother, queen, crone), masculine-feminine balancing, trance work on balancing of power and beauty and so forth.

These rituals also facilitate our awareness of archetypal forces -- instinctive and universal elements manifesting from the collective unconscious.   These universal themes are found in fairy tales, mythological narratives, movies and even in our dreams. Evoking these psychic energies in a ritual setting enables women to re-affirm missing parts of their own psyches.   Sometimes our groups simply focus on more awareness of the elements (fire, and/or earth, air, water).

Focusing on an element in ritual can deepen their relationship with nature.   For example, in May of 2001 I went with a group to Israel. This small piece of land holds an incredible display of history. One can stand in an ancient Roman cave dedicated to the pagan god Pan, visit honored Jewish, Christian and Muslim sites. And enter first excavations of ancient Canaanite sites, which honor the Goddess.

Separating from the group, I eagerly climbed down into a small hole leading down to a cave-like space where I could see the beginning excavations of perfectly formed steps leading down into what would have been an ancient Canaanite city. I entered into silent meditation. Soon thereafter, I experienced what I felt to be a "fire from underneath." This inner experience is difficult to explain in ordinary language. This power, present and ancient, emanated from a deep feminine source. After returning to the United States I decided that "fire" would be the focal

157

point of our next ritual group.

Twenty women sit in a circle on the ground as the ritual begins. We evoke the elements and repeat the affirmation of the beauty and power of Mother Earth. The trance ritual begins with actual fire in the center of the circle and inner, evocative images of fire. . . the attributes *inspiration, transformation.* I shape a ball of fire with inner eyes and hands. This ball of fire passes to the next woman, who then passes it to the next. We all sense this ball getting larger and larger as it passes around the circle. When it returns to me, I release it to the center of the circle.

Each of us experienced blessing from the fire ball—something akin to being bathed in a warm kindness. Typically, one doesn't think of "fire" as emanating "kindness," but we all shared this similar awareness. The fire-ball provided both individual and shared awareness. It helped our community of women to move past issues of mistrust and to open our hearts to one another.

Many women are somewhat untrusting of one another, influenced by a few thousand years of being deemed "inferior" beings. Think of the erroneous interpretation of Eve being created from Adam's rib. The original understanding (in Sumerian) can be translated as *She who gives life.* When a human being is prevented from expressing one's self in the world (creatively, for example), mistrust and hidden aggression lurk in the background, projected onto mothers, sisters, female friends. Group rituals for feminine expression and being help to heal these ancient wounds, both internal and external.

Rituals to help strengthen communal bonds are surely needed throughout the world, especially crucial to include the feminine and our connectedness to Mother Earth. As men recognize their inner feminine, and welcome women as an equal presence in the world, all will change for the better. As women reclaim their spirits and their bodies, they can stand in partnership. In unison we can heal the planet and redeem humanity. Sky and earth reunited.

3

TRANSFORMATIVE EXPERIENCES WITH RITUAL

ONE NIGHT IN BANGKOK: BURNING MAN REFLECTIONS

MICHAEL CARROLL

I'M TRAPPED, CRAWLING HEAD FIRST THROUGH A NARROW PASSAGEWAY that seems to be getting tighter and tighter as I inch forward. I'm not sure where I am or what will be waiting for me if I can get out of this tunnel. Excitement turns to anxiety, my breathing speeds up and my heart starts beating like a bass drum as I struggle through the cramped darkness. Finally, I see some light breaking through a vertical slit ahead of me. I hear a familiar voice calling out, but I can't quite decipher the message. "What?!" I yell. My friend Tim responds, "Don't forget to kiss the clitoris on your way out!" "Ah-ha!" It all dawns on me as I pull myself through the flaps of a gigantic vagina, constructed of wood, carpet, etc., and lay a big wet one on the clit. And there I stand on the other side, born anew into the wonderful world of Burning Man.

Past the lips of the vagina, there's a dance party going on inside a wooden fort. The artificial birth canal is the entrance to the party. A DJ hovers in the watchtower up above, spinning a most fitting song for my entrance into this new land and life:

One night in Bangkok and the world's your oyster
The bars are temples but the pearls ain't free
You'll find a god in every golden cloister

And if you're lucky then the god's a she
I can feel an angel sliding up to me
    (One Night in Bangkok, Benny Anderson, Tim Rice, & Bjsrn Ulvaeus)

"What the hell is going on here? Where am I? How did I get here?" I wonder, as I stand giggling in awe, trying to take it all in. Just a few days before I was flying from Chicago to San Francisco for a much needed vacation. San Francisco was a haze, as San Francisco tends to be. Then this morning I drove up to the Burn with my friend Tim and two buddies of his, all of us Burning Man rookies, not really sure what we were getting into. We had heard stories, seen pictures. It would be hot. There would be lots of topless women. Drugs and dancing. Freaks getting weird. What more could you need? Apparently at the end of it all there is supposed to be a giant wooden statue of a man that gets burned down, hence the name, "Burning Man."

We pulled in under the cover of darkness, gazing at the strange scene developing all around us. A temporary city constructed from scratch in the middle of a Nevada desert, just past Nowheretown, USA. Around 30,000 people set up camp, trucking in U-hauls, RV's, and semi's filled with sound-systems, giant tents, art pieces, and various amusements, plus all the food, drink, and supplies they'll need to survive in this harsh climate for about a week. This little city is more than a little different from any other city you may have encountered. The normal rules don't apply here.

Even now, it's still hard to put a finger on exactly what Burning Man is, or even what it isn't. With such a wide variety of experiences to be had, I imagine everyone who attends would describe it differently. For some it's a sacred pilgrimage, the culmination of an entire year of preparation, and a chance to express and explore their soul. For others, it's the height of decadence, a chance to shed all inhibitions, express oneself creatively, and dabble in the taboos of our dominant culture, particularly drugs and sex. For most, its probably somewhere in between the sacred and profane. But after a few days in the desert, with all the chaos swirling around you, the profane may become sacred, and vice versa. With my new post-Burn perspective, I'm quite sure that celebrating life, partying as hard as you can, joyously and deviously expressing yourself, shedding your inhibitions and persona, sharing this experience with others in community, and just plain getting your ya-ya's out is the most sacred thing one can do.

I'm not sure what all the necessary components of a ritual are, but I think Burning Man can be seen as the ultimate post-modern do-it-yourself ritual. There is a smorgasbord of activities to partake in, so that everyone tailors their experience to suit their needs, delights, and interests. People have asked me what Burning Man is all about, and in the past I've described it as a cross between the parking lot scene at a Grateful Dead show, a giant rave, a post-apocalyptic Road Warrior landscape, and an adult amusement park. Those are my reference points anyway. To some they might do little to relate the nature of the experience, so I'll do my best to describe, point-by-point, what went down in the desert.

Step 1: Apply sunscreen. The sun and sand are everywhere, you can't escape them, so you must submit to the will of the harsh desert climate. Reapply the sunscreen continuously and generously, strap on your sunglasses, and keep a bandana over your face to keep the dust out. Drink lots of water, as well as any other beverages you need to get you through the night. These are the habitual, as opposed to the ritual, necessities of Burning Man that quickly become second nature.

Step 2: Bring a bike, and ride off into the sunset. My crew brought a few pawnshop dirt bikes, just like the kind I had when I was 10, which had the effect of transporting my consciousness back to that age of innocence and wonder. We rode across the desert like a gang of marauders, ready to take on the new world, and see what it had in store for us, just like when we were kids.

Step 3: Reapply sunscreen.

Step 4: Dance on top of a pillar with half-naked women. Pick your jaw up off the floor.

Step 5: Stick your head up the ass of a gigantic two-story tall homemade goat. Speak to the strange men inside the belly of the goat. Ask them where you can find god in the desert, and eat the Cheeto they put on your tongue. Pull your head out of the goat's ass, and stumble away dazed and confused.

Step 6: Did I mention the sunscreen?

Step 7: Confess to your friends that the goat, and the guys inside, freaked you out. Laugh and smile till it hurts, as they tell you the same. Plot to steal a car and crash it into the goat, and imagine watching the goat go up in flames.

Step 8: Get out of the way of the dragon! There's a giant metal dragon coming your way, breathing fire, and the driver is pissed that your crew is blocking its path. It eats hippies for breakfast, so you better think fast or you'll soon find yourself in the belly of the beast.

Step 9: In the midst of all the chaos swirling round, a hush will overcome you as you encounter the Temple of Sacred Tears. A giant ornate wooden structure in the middle of the desert, ineffable, the most beautiful structure this side of Gaudi's La Sagrada Familia. A moment of reflection, as you take in the beauty of this building dedicated to suicide victims. There are wooden blocks for you to write down prayers, or the names of the departed. This is a holy place, with a feeling of reverence. At the end of the festival, all of this will be burned to the ground.

Step 10: Sunscreen anyone?

Step 11: Return to your camp to recharge. Burning Man can be both physically and mentally exhausting, with the intense climate, plus all the chaotic festivities. Your campmates are like-minded in feelings of exhaustion. A brief return to normalcy is needed, so Classic Rock Happy Hour is spontaneously thought up. Beers are cracked open as you kick back in a comfy chair, and Tom Petty's *American Girl* blares out of the speakers. Naked women are bathing in a pool set up across the street, and you can't look away. Everything in the universe is exactly as it should be. You are smiling.

Well she was an American girl
Raised on promises
She couldn't help thinkin' that there
Was a little more to life
Somewhere else
After all it was a great big world

With lots of places to run to
Yeah, and if she had to die
Tryin' she had one little promise
She was gonna keep

(American Girl, Tom Petty & The Heartbreakers)

Step 12: Your peace is disturbed, as you notice a strange commotion headed your way. A group of naked people, bodies painted completely red, are chasing down a poor soul. They pick him up, and start to carry him off. As you attempt to take a picture of this bizarre scene they spot you and start pointing in your direction. You better high tail it out of there. They're coming for you.

Step 13: In your escape from the red people, you stumble across a geodesic dome, with triangular spikes in an arc around the top. You have just encountered Camp Boognish, named for the band Ween's morally ambiguous god, the Boognish, both god and Satan rolled into one. Inside the dome Ween is blaring, naturally, so you go check it out. It's empty, except for a man with pink hair. He tells you his name is Pink Money. He has come to Burning Man to get married in the desert. You congratulate him, tell him about the two Ween shows you just saw in San Francisco, and how you were pleasantly surprised to find Camp Boognish. You invite him back to your camp, Camp Juicy, for a drink.

Step 14: On the way back to Camp Juicy, you spot a green shack in the distance. Spray painted on the side is "Camp Skynyrd." A scantily clad woman is leaning in the doorway. This shack could just as easily be a roadhouse in Alabama, but it's not out of place at Burning Man. You're curious who this woman is, and what's inside the shack, but you have to get back to Camp Juicy.

Step 15: Oh shit! I forgot the sunscreen!

Step 16: Why call it Camp Juicy, you ask? The collective I'm camping with has brought several hundred pounds of frozen fruit, many bottles of liquor, and blenders. Someone even managed to procure a license to operate a kitchen. We make frozen fruit drinks, throw a party, and hand them out to anyone who shows up. This is how the economy of Burning

Man works. There is no buying or selling, or even bartering. It is a gift-based economy. People give things away. If you need something, you ask if you can have it. Sometimes you will be told no, but usually yes. Sometimes you will be asked to perform a service in return. This is such a dramatic departure from American culture that it takes some getting used to. Once you get the idea, you realize it's like a non-stop Christmas, except you get to play the role of both the kids and Santa. Not bad.

Step 17: Dusk. The witching hour. The gloaming. Things are starting to get weird, as if they weren't weird enough yet. You can hear howling out in the desert. Music is coming from all directions. You're excited and apprehensive at the same time. If you've brought any mind-altering substances, and haven't ingested them yet, now would be the time

Step 18: A giant ark is passing by, so you climb on in for a spin around the desert. Actually it's a converted school bus, but your legs are a little wobbly, your stomach a little queasy, and damn if you don't feel like you're on a ship. Ahoy!

Step 19: The first stop of the evening is a dance party. The music is bumping, but the few people inside are all sitting on the side like wallflowers. Your crew is feeling it, and you're all out on the dance floor doing the Charleston, running man, and whatever other dance moves you can remember. The DJ's are loving it, and respond in kind. The wallflowers are brought to life, and join the fun. And just as quickly as you've arrived, its time to leave. On to the next one.

Step 20: Crawl through a vagina and be born into a new world and new person. One of the ultimate symbolic experiences, with others still to come. As a wise man once told me in broken English, "the night, it is like a little baby."

Step 21: Marvel at the giant green laser beam emanating from a neon Mayan temple, shooting across the entire desert, off into the mountains in the distance. Walk under the laser; follow it to see where it leads.

Step 22: Apparently you weren't the only person following the laser, as you stumble across a man rolling in the desert sand, laughing. You say hello, and he smiles back at you with pupils as big as silver dollars. You ask him if he's ok, and he just laughs and falls down. There's nothing you can do for him. Either he's a raving lunatic, or he's found the secret of life, or both. You wish him good luck, and continue on your way; you've got a laser to follow.

Step 23: Scattered along the path of the laser are many strange occurrences in the desert. They're art installations of various size and variety that people have been working on all year, brought out, and constructed in the desert. Some are meant to be pondered, others interacted with. I can't really do them justice, and my memory is quite likely distorted, but examples can be viewed at HYPERLINK www.burningman.com.

Step 24: The laser leads you to a large wooden 2-story building. You enter, and quickly find yourself in a maze, winding down passages, running into dead ends, going through doorways in the dark. You get separated from your crew, and somehow wind up on the second floor by yourself. There's a fire pole on the side of the building. The night has been long and your senses are distorted, so you decide to get out of this madhouse and slide down the pole. Your friends were looking for you, and you carry on. The laser beckons.

Step 25: A man asks you if you have any shrooms (a.k.a. "magic mushrooms"). He looks like a narc, so you tell him "no." He says, "thanks anyway," and hands you a nice homemade Burning Man sticker that will be attached to your coffee table for years to come. You feel bad for thinking he was a narc.

Step 26: The laser leads you further out in the desert, and back to your childhood, as you encounter several games from your youth. The games aren't the normal size though, as they're built to Alice in Wonderland scale. A four-foot tall Connect Four set. A six-foot long Shoot the Moon, etc. You don't feel like a child. You are a child.

Step 27: Child's play is over. There is a sinister side to the desert also. You encounter a large dome, just a naked metal frame. Inside two bungee cords are attached to the top, and combatants swing from either side of the of the dome and hit each other with padded bats. Spectators dangle from the outside of the dome to observe the potential danger within. Brave souls line up to take their turn, as the leather-clad man with the Mohawk prepares them for battle. Chants of "two men enter, one man leaves" erupt through the crowd. Burning Man is not all peace, love, and sunshine.

Step 28: You've lost track of the laser now and are in the open desert. Big mistake. A sandstorm whips up, and you can't see a foot in front of your face. You wander aimlessly for what seems like hours, stumbling across other lost souls, and encountering art installations that appear seemingly out of thin air. Finally, the storm dies down. You're exhausted, and can barely stay on your feet. But as the man said, you're wasted and you can't find your way home. Burning Man is a city, and if you lose your way you'll be in for a long night. But truly, all who wander are not lost, and you come across a dapper gentleman in suit and top hat. You ask him for directions, and he grins like a Cheshire cat. He's told this tale before, and he does it in style. He shows you the simple way to get your bearings straight if lost, with the Burning Man statue in the middle of the desert city acting as the compass. You're glad you got lost, as it gave you the opportunity to interact with this character, whose class, impeccable style, charisma, and generosity embodies the Burning Man ethic.

Step 29: You stumble back into camp, and reconvene with a few friends who are off to one final party of the night. You can't resist. You come upon a smallish tent, that from the looks of it is about to explode. It's filled to the gills with gyrating bodies. There's a band onstage throwing it down hard, fast, and heavy; a mini P-Funk orchestra, horn section and all, blaring away. The trumpet player is going off. The music is building and building to peak after peak. Hands are up in the air. Everyone is screaming at the top of their lungs. The trumpet player is walking the tightrope, hanging on for dear life, letting it all hang out, holding it for an eternity, then hitting that one final note causing the collective third eye of all in attendance to explode. Thirty seconds after you entered, its all over, the greatest 30 seconds of your life, you're quite sure.

Step 30: Hey Mr. Tambourine man, play a song for me. You've given all you can, experienced more than you can digest, and fall asleep before your head hits the pillow. Sleep for two hours, wake up, and do it all over again.

Yes, to dance beneath the diamond sky with one hand waving free
Silhouetted by the sea, circled by the circus sands
With all memory and fate driven deep beneath the waves
Let me forget about today until tomorrow.

(Mr. *Tambourine Man,* Bob Dylan)

After a few days, I started to get the hang of it. Initially I found myself hesitant and overwhelmed by everything that was going on around me, and the drastic departure it all was from the reality I was used to. Eventually I was able to shift from the role of observer to participant. At Burning Man, humans are the art pieces. Truly a transpersonal festival, Burning Man gives the opportunity to shed the persona that you present to the world, and express your true self. Or try on different selves and see what you like. There is no right or wrong way to be, so the shadow can come out to play. Burning Man operates on multiple levels, showing us what is possible for each of us individually, as well as collectively, within American culture and the human. It opens the door, and allows you to peek inside. Maybe you see how wrong you've been living your life, and how screwed up American culture is. But it gives you hope, because you can see what's possible. That eternal dream of personal liberation and communal living is realized every year for a few days. Hope.

Everyone at Burning Man realizes this. And on the final night, 30,000 participants stand in a circle around the Man, a 100-foot tall wooden statue of a man. He has a skeletal frame of neon lights. His arms, which had been down by his side, are now reaching up to the sky. He stands at the center of the desert city, and the center of your experience. Night falls, and the previous insanity is taken to a whole new level. A band behind you is playing a variety of appropriate tunes, including *Disco Inferno* by the Tramps, *Burning Down the House* by the Talking Heads, and *Fire*, by Jimi Hendrix. "*Let me stand next to your fire/ motherfuckin fire!*" People are decked out in their finest threads. Others are running around screaming. Fire dancers are twirling their flames. The energy is building. And then, BOOM! Fireworks are set off from the Man, and he is ablaze. He catches fire fast, and it spreads quickly to his head. Everyone is howling. The heat is building. Hands are thrown up in the air. One arm on the Man falls. Then the man topples over. There is a great rush. You come within 20 yards of the Man, and the heat is intense. Hotter than anything you've ever felt. People are going berserk, ripping their clothes off and throwing them into the fire. The circle starts moving clockwise around the flaming remains of the Man. 30,000 people running in a gigantic clusterfuck. It's both exhilarating and frightening, as the heat and sea of people is overwhelming. You hang on for as long as you can, but you can take no more and you retreat. You take a few steps back, as bliss overtakes you. How is this possible? What is this? You can't consciously make sense of it all, yet it makes perfect sense. This is how rituals, and their symbols, operate: on an unconscious level. The cleansing fire, burning the past and all of its attachments away. Burning away your past self, your previous conceptions of humanity, and even the festival experience itself. A destructive act of creation. Killing the past, to allow for a new future. Don't look back.

We shall not cease from exploration
And the end of all our exploring
Will be to arrive where we started
And know the place for the first time.

(*Four Quartets, T. S. Elliot*)

And so I returned to the world, to Chicago, to my job, to my friends and family. But I wasn't the same person, and I saw the world with new eyes. The Burning Man ritual, and all of the symbols, take you on a journey to the desert, away from the world. But more importantly, as you're on this outer journey in this peculiar land with its experiences and symbolic content, a corresponding inner journey is taking place. All true rituals are the outer representations of inner processes of transformation. Burning Man symbolizes and conjures up the journey to a strange a challenging place, filled with mysteries, wonders, fears, and bizarre characters, all inside yourself. Analogues to many of the experiences I had in the desert, and people I encountered, can be found in fairytales and myths told since the beginning of time. The archetypal Hero's Journey.

And it is with these new eyes that I saw the world one week later, on the morning of September 11, 2001. I arrived at work just after the first plane hit the Twin Towers, and my coworkers couldn't believe what was happening. I acted shocked, but all I could think was "of course!" This was bound to happen. We live our lives so out of touch with ourselves, the people we know, other cultures, and the earth, striving after purpose-less goals, mindlessly going through the motions, the truth of our human-ity buried so deep down inside, that this was bound to happen.

It isn't until now that I realize: in 9/11 the archetypal Burning Man experience was being created in the real world, the symbols coming to life, albeit on a disturbing and drastic level. The Twin Towers, just like the Man, were set ablaze by people fed up with American culture, re-pressed by their own cultures, and striving for personal and spiritual free-dom. And just as we danced around the remnants of the Man with both feelings of fear and bliss, people in far away lands were out dancing in the streets as the World Trade Center crumbled to the ground. It seems strange that these two profound experiences of mine, Burning Man and 9/11, occurred within a week of each other. Maybe Burning Man pre-pared me for what was to come.

Maybe the sun will shine today
The clouds will blow away
Maybe I won't feel so afraid
I will try to understand
Everything has its plan
Either way
(Either Way, Jeff Tweedy & Wilco)

My coworkers went home that morning on 9/11. I kept on working, I can't say why. Maybe I didn't want to give in to the fear. Maybe I just had some work I wanted to get done. I called my future wife and told her I loved her, and then drove off to an adult day care in a lower income area of Chicago. I had some cognitive testing to do with Alzheimer's patients. These people had lived hard, and been witness to some of the great tragedies of humanity: wars, racism, the bomb. Now for the most part they were oblivious to what had happened that morning. Those who could smiled and joked around. We bounced a ball around the room, did some exercises, and they answered my questions. For them it was just another day.

What does it all mean? Even after writing all this, I still can't quite say. Hopefully the mysteries of Burning Man will continue to inform my life all the way, and to the end. I don't think it's possible to understand a ritual from the intellectual perspective of our normal waking consciousness. If we could, maybe it would rob rituals of their mystery and magic. So I feel it is fitting to end this piece by paying tribute to the wisdom of a man who died on the day this story was conceived, 4/11/2007. Life and all its wonders and tragedies may make little sense, but in the immortal words of Kurt Vonnegut: "... *trust me on the Sunscreen.*"

And "*So it goes...*"

UNEXPECTED TRANSFORMATION

COLETTE FLEURIDAS

THE WORD "RITUAL" BRINGS UP LESS THAN POSITIVE ASSOCIATIONS FOR me, in general. I do not enjoy staged or repetitive rituals, and very few have been meaningful or inspiring to me. Curiosity has motivated me to investigate many forms of ritual, but I prefer to avoid formal secular or religious ceremonies. When my partner and I co-created a very small but lovely wedding in the woods, where very little was said or done.

I have, however, been very interested in what generates and supports transformation. The spontaneous and sometimes unexpected opening of my body-heart-mind, whether I am alone in nature or in other sacred and/or social settings, has been the primary source of my transformative experiences. This has rarely occurred while participating in staged, ritualized performances. Exceptions are most apt to happen if I am with a community that is alive, aware, present, engaged, and free to be genuine and spontaneous. Twenty years ago, I was invited to into a multi-tribal Native American community; the transformative effects of some of their rituals surprised me. Inspired by their traditions, I entered into an experience that dramatically changed my sense of self and of Spirit.

The most meaningful ritualized ceremony in this particular community was the Native American Long Dance celebration. Approximately 60 men, women, and children from across North America came together on each equinox and solstice, for three or four days, to camp in a beautiful, remote location in the Utah wilderness. We gathered to fast and pray, to sing and chant, to drum and dance, to be still and silent, to welcome the next phase of the Earth's cycle around the sun, to listen to the inner call of the Great Spirit and of one's ancestors, and to support each of our personal and collective intentions for the coming season. Elders from the First Nations of the North West Coast-Coast Salish peoples; the local medicine men from the Ute, Paiute, and Shoshone tribes; the shaman from the Northeast; and Grandmother from the Hopi Nation, as well as others, worked together to support our collective purpose. They guided us through the opening ceremonies, the sweat lodges at dusk, the ritualized river cleanses at dawn, the 24 hour prayerful and sacrificial dance through the day and night, the peace pipe ceremony, and the closing rituals.

For many of us from Euro-American heritages, the rituals, the dances, the chants, and the approach to the Holy were different than what we had learned from our elders. However, most of us felt our deep inner union with and appreciation for Nature, our innate relationship with all the beings that live upon this planet, and our collective responsibility to live wisely, in respect and care for all manifestations of Spirit. The principles and practices of these Native teachers enriched my spirituality with a renewed openness to the varieties of spiritual experience within nature and within the self.

My spiritual interests began to emerge slowly in a curious childhood. I was not reared in religious dogma and was free to be immersed in the awe of the divine presence of Nature. From early adolescence, onward, my spiritual development expanded through many stages: through the intellectual yearnings of youth, when I experienced a deep devotional desire to know intimately the God of the Judaeo-Christians; through the silent centering prayer of the West in my young 20s, to know Truth inside myself; and into mid-adulthood, through the mindful meditation and self-inquiry practices of the East, to experience the Absolute. I was both skeptical of and curious about the beliefs and spiritual practices of this diverse Native American community. Within a few hours of participating in the opening ceremonies of the Long Dance, my body-mind-heart opened as I tasted the spiritual essence of Nature. Thus, with community, through ritual, and into nature I ventured, to learn more about self, the interconnection of all beings, and the Ultimate.

During this time, I learned about other American Indian ritualized opportunities to experience Truth in many forms. Vision quests, once mostly unknown in the West, became more popular in the United States in the later part of the 1900s. Historically, in some native tribes, adolescents made their way into adulthood through their own vision quests; this quest was usually a several day journey, alone, in nature and into the spiritual realms acknowledged by that tribal community. The intent was to quest for a vision or for a deeper understanding of the adolescents' personal significance. Often, this solo journey provided them with an opportunity to discover their totem or spiritual/animal guides, who would assist them to learn more specifically about their life purpose and how to live in wisdom on the earth. Another central and paradoxical feature of spending several days alone in nature was the profound experience of their inner aloneness paired with a deeper knowing of their interdependent relationship with All That Is.

Back in the summer of 1987, four of us decided to spend a few days camping in a remote wilderness area in Southern Utah. My partner and I, and another couple to whom we were very close, were eager to support each other to go on our own individual vision quests. Responsibility for children and work limited our excursion to a weekend. As I write this memoire, I recall that I kept a journal at that time. After skimming through the words written almost twenty years ago by a woman (whom I remember but no longer identify as myself), I found this entry (July 12, 1987) that describes what I wish to share, my first experience of a vision quest:

Spent the weekend camping . . . the four of us in the Capitol Reef area . . . earthy colors, juniper, spruce, yellow wild flowers, rabbits, snakes, lizards . . . incredibly beautiful. Friday night, we talked late into the night by the camp fire, . . . full moon, prayers and songs to the four directions, welcoming the spirits . . . The sky and earth kissed in perfect beauty . . . We greeted dawn with ritual songs and prayers for the day, and each took off, alone, on our vision quests. Saturday was a difficult day for me. My intent was to continue the beautiful visionary work that I had begun to explore the weeks before . . . At dawn, I took off from the campsite and hiked along the ridge above a canyon . . . I walked with tremendous deter-mination, asking [the Great Spirit and spiritual guides] for insight, reve-lation, knowledge, wisdom, and contact, contact with something outside of myself – some sign – some assurance that I am not creating my own reality apart from a Real reality, from Truth. I longed deeply for such; [given my recent influence from the Native tradition], simple signs would satisfy, such as the visitation of a butterfly, or a rabbit to sit and look at me and not run away. (I thought that the butterfly was too difficult to manifest, since I hadn't seen any in this arid place, but there were a few rabbits. However, then I thought that my plea was altogether ridiculous.)

I sat down [on the rocky ledge overlooking the shallow canyon].
I waited.
[hours passed]
I felt no sense of Spirit.
I felt no sense of God, nor even the love, comfort, tingling sensations,
and gentle vibrations that usually welled up from inside me
whenever I meditated or prayed.

I only felt despair and emptiness, nothingness.
I wondered, perhaps there is only nothingness beyond this reality;
perhaps there is only death and physical erosion into the earth and gasses,
a destiny without purpose or identity.
I began to believe this quite strongly and felt deep despair;
I lost all motivation . . . to return to be with the others,
and to continue with my work as a therapist.

As I sat, I felt and saw my body dying,
decaying quickly in the dry heat;
tears streamed down my checks
until I felt my flesh disappear and
my bones crumble into dust.
I saw the tiny white particles blow away into nothingness.

My consciousness remained without form.
I felt forsaken – my beliefs had failed me – my God . . .
I remembered Jesus's words and pondered his experience of death,
especially if he believed that he would never die . . .
It helped me, a little, to recall this.

Slowly, hours later, the sun's rays no longer visible,
I had gained enough energy to return to camp,
very slowly,
despairing, with no belief, no hope,
(or little hope).
I did have the knowledge of the love that I shared with my friends and family,
and I longed for their love,
but, otherwise, I had lost my sense of purpose,
sense of being,
sense of power, of creativity, of direction, of healing, of energy, of spirit
[and of optimism, all prevalent in my day-to-day life up until that day];
now these experiences of being were a doubted memory.

My girlfriend greeted me with the power and exuberance gained during her inner journey, which she shared with me as we lay on the quilt by the campfire. It was comforting to learn of her vision, to feel her faith and love, and to hear her insights about her life unfolding. My other friend and I did not connect deeply, and it was difficult for my partner to understand what I was experiencing, especially since I did not share the depth of the transformation with him. I wondered if I would ever feel the energy of spirit in my body again . . . perhaps, after some rest. The four of us spent the next day, Sunday, hiking and sharing stories about our time alone. At the end of the day, just prior to leaving the camp, I saw a white butterfly . . . and as we pulled out in our jeep, I saw a rabbit, a cottontail, hop to the side of the road and sit and stare at me as we drove away. I wondered if those were the simple signs that I had sought.

I skim through the rest of the journal to see if what I remember about this turning point is validated in my writings from that time. What I recall is that, after my vision quest, I experienced myself differently in relation to spiritual knowing and faith. I became deeply uncertain about the meaning of all my previous and profound spiritual experiences and beliefs. However, I was clear about the continuing value of love, goodness, beauty, and truthfulness. Although I did journal about other spiritual realizations and experiences, I wrote this, a couple months later:

Sadness,
never so constant,
never so present,
never so profound,
never so pervasive;
I do not want you to be wiped away as a tear.

Sadness, here.
Teach me your lesson,
your power,
your meaning,
your call.
Sadness, anger, lack of trust, despair, hopelessness:
I do not ask to see your beauty but only to stay with your essence.

It is the only thing that feels true, right now,
not because I can hope for it to lead to something better,
although I know that it may; I also know that it may not.
But right now, sadness feels more real and honest than any
other Way of Being.

The journal also contains entries about my three young children, their personalities budding forth beautifully, their birthdays, and their new adventures. I also wrote about work and job transitions (I left a community counseling center to become the clinical director of a 40-bed inpatient treatment center for Native Americans and prison diversion clients). I grappled with the changes in my closest friendships and described the continuing passion in my marriage. However, I was changing. Other friends noticed that I was no longer my "normal" energetic, joyful, optimistic self. I had shared my experience with a few close friends and had generated numerous possible explanations for what had occurred. I continued to work within the Native community for my own healing and spiritual insights. I also had support and inspiration from the small transpersonal psychology community in Salt Lake City. Then a month after the fall equinox, and participating in the three-day Long Dance ceremony in Southern Utah, I wrote in my journal:

> *I want to go deeper, now.*
> *I weave in and out of believing,*
> *in and out of hoping,*
> *in and out of desiring to know,*
> *and, usually,*
> *I weave in.*
> *I feel unconnected, right now, except, of course, to my children.*
> *I feel like I haven't found what I am looking for –*
> *and often wonder if I ever will*
> *or if "it" even exists.*

My search for spiritual truth began in my early teens, when I had a heart-opening spiritual experience while alone, in nature. After a year or two of exploring different faith communities, I dove whole heartedly into charismatic Christianity: the trust, love and joy of the youthful devotional community were inspiring to me. After a couple of years, at age 17, I entered college to study religion (and went on to earn a master's degree at a seminary); I became a member of a thriving spiritual community in Southern California that engaged in esoteric practices similar to those described in the Book of Acts in the New Testament. The sincerity, genuineness, and intelligence of the majority of those in this group were attractive. I had a very committed daily prayer life and devotional practice, as well as an intellectual thirst for truth in all its manifestations. By my early-twenties, after reading texts from other spiritual traditions as well as learning Biblical Greek, some Hebrew, exegetical skills to interpret the Bible, and Judaeo-Christian history, I could no longer call myself a Christian. I had learned too much about this and other religions, and about the insights and experiences of mystics across traditions, to limit myself to one faith.

It was challenging on many levels for me to leave the Christian community that had been my extended family for almost a decade. I began to explore the quieter paths into truth through meditative sitting with the local, open-minded Quaker community and with the Zen Buddhists, who had a small sangha in Iowa City. While I was attending graduate school at the university to earn my doctorate in counseling and human development, I struggled with the constructs of the divine within and the god(s) outside of the self. Learning about the theories and research that attempt to foster a greater understanding of the human psyche was fascinating, and assisted me to gain some perspective about religious faith and spiritual experience.

A few years later, while doing my clinical internship in Utah, I was invited to participate in the Native American Long Dance ceremonies; I began to study Indigenous spiritual practices, beliefs, and values. I deeply appreciated the emphasis of the Native people on our inherent interconnection with all that exists. Central to their faith and prayer was the acknowledgment that all people, all beings, and all elements are inter-related and, ultimately, One. Incorporating these values into my unfolding spiritual conceptualizations filled me with a deep sense of social and environmental responsibility for the well being of our planet and for all who dwell upon her.

What a mystery this was for me, to embark upon a vision quest with an intent to deepen my knowledge of the Sacred and of myself, and to experience a kind of death, a total nothingness, an absence of spirit, and to crawl back from the edge of nature's abyss into my humanity with despair and hopelessness. For the first time in my life, I sensed that I understood some (though not all) of the physical and psychological aspects of the chronic depression felt by many of my clients.

A couple of years passed, and the impact of my vision quest continued to influence me. I left Utah to take an academic position in a rural community in Northern California. Although I loved teaching at a state university, my health had been challenged for months. After a series of blood tests from my medical doctor, and ruling out known conditions that would explain the fatigue and low grade fevers that I felt most afternoons and evenings, I had sought the help of a naturopathic physician and of an acupuncturist. Their herbal remedies were helpful, as well as their questions: When did I first recall feeling this way? I remembered back to the day when I sat in silence and beauty, on the canyon ridge in the wilderness, when I entered into this deep, evolving sadness.

Years passed again and I was at a personal growth workshop in Hawaii with my partner. At the end of several days of participating in various spiritual and psychological activities, we were invited to pair up into dyads and to participate in a ritual. We were instructed to journey back in time to a challenging experience that still had an impact on us. Then we were invited to bring this experience into the present, somatically and with an open heart. I partnered with my mate and, after his impactful experience, it was my turn. I chose to focus on my vision quest from nine years earlier. Through the guidance of the facilitator and with the support of my partner, I lay on my back and began the ritual. In my body-heart-mind, I relived the journey into the desert and to the canyon ridge, where I began my meditation. As prompted, I verbalized each of the details that I recalled: the physical experience of gradually losing my vitality; my breath becoming stiller and less apparent; the vision of my body decaying and of my bones blowing away in the wind; no sense of self other than a witness; the consideration that this final experience is our only destiny; and the emotional despair that followed. Then my partner invited me to bring this memory into the present moment energetically, breathing fully, and keeping all parts of myself open and aware.

With the facilitator's guidance, I could feel the stillness of death in my body, once again, and my bones decaying and turning to dust. This time, however, as I shared my experience moment by moment, rather than blowing away, the bone-dust twirled above me in a stream of gold light. The dust sparkled brilliantly as light-reflecting particles of gold spiraling up into the sky from my being. My body began to shiver and shake, even though the temperature of the room was quite warm. Bliss filled me and tears streamed down my checks uncontrollably as I lay in silence, shivering in delight. After an unknown passage of time, I was assisted to walk out doors and, for over an hour, I was in this state. Hours and days passed, but the feeling of bliss and aliveness remained. Sadness was still available, but no longer prevalent. The spiritual joy and psychological optimism, which were dominant in my life before my vision quest, now returned as mysteriously as they had left.

The Shaman with the Flashing Lights

Fred Alan Wolf

My earlier time with Ed McGaa had taught me something about the Sioux Indians. They always keep their word. Although my first encounter with Doug was less than I had expected, I knew that Paul would return. So about seven that evening, as dusk rapidly approached, I went outside of my apartment, and there Paul was, sitting in his pickup truck. Sitting next to him was a man with a natty brown shirt on. He was wearing a naval sea captain's cap. It even said "captain" on the brim. I laughed at that and I walked over to see who this was. It was Doug, the shaman. He was all cleaned up. He was wearing clean clothes and he had shaved. He also smelled high of Brut, the men's cologne.

I was amazed at his transformation. He then wanted to talk with one of the nurses in the hospital. I followed Doug and Paul into the emergency room and introduced him to a nurse named Mary that I met earlier. Well, Mary recognized him. Seeing that the nurse he wanted to meet was not there, Doug asked for a telephone, and finding out where it was, he left me standing with Mary. Mary pulled me by the elbow to a corner of the room. She whispered to me, "You better watch out for him."

I said, "Why?"

"Because he's drunk."

I knew from his behavior that he wasn't drunk. But I then realized why Mary believed he was. It was the Brut. He had smeared it all over his body, and it made him smell of alcholol.

I then realized that I may be dealing with a *Heyokah*, a trickster-shaman. I realized that he probably wasn't even drunk when I met him that morning, he just smelled high of Brut.

Doug returned and we walked outside. Doug approached me and began acting as if he were drunk. He asked me if I could help him out with some money. I looked at him, and, again, he appeared as if he were a bum. I realized that Doug was getting my emotions all upset. He was pushing all of my buttons. I didn't even realize that until several days later. Somehow Doug knew just what my buttons were. And money was definitely one of my buttons. He knew just what to say to upset me. But how could he know?

I then realized that Doug had quite a lot of shamanic power, not only because of his abilities to push my emotional buttons but also to play the tragic clown role so well.

Soon we left the compound. I followed them in their pickup back through a windstorm in the plains. It was dusty and blowing a hot wind, as the sun was beginning to set. I could barely see their truck ahead of me, the dust storm was so bad. Yet, I managed to follow Paul and Doug in their pickup back along the main road threading through the reservation, toward the town of Oglala. We soon reached a dirt road leading off toward the left of the main road, leading to a house up toward the hills of the badlands of South Dakota. With each mile, I found myself growing more and more suspicious. As we left the main road, it was getting darker and darker, and at the same time more and more brush and plant life, shrubs and trees appeared to be looming around me. I was becoming frightened, and I felt as if I were taking a journey into the darkness of my soul.

We finally arrived at a small house nestled against the foothills. It was very dark now. There are no street lights anywhere on the reservation except near the hospital compound.

I walked into the house. There were a number of people assembled. Against one side of the living room nestled a small wood stove. There was no other heating available. The windows were totally covered with blankets and curtains. Folding chairs were arranged along three sides of the room, making a square with one side missing. I noticed that the walls were colored pink. I also noticed that every mirror in the house as covered. My fear began to grow.

Sitting were three Indian women. I then asked one of the women about the ceremony. "Is this going to be a Yuwipi ceremony?" I wondered aloud. She said, "No, it's a thanksgiving ceremony for Paul." I later found out that this was called an *Olowonpi* ceremony. All of the lights in the house would be turned out, as in a Yuwipi, making the room as dark as possible. Certainly spirits would come. I would see flashing of lights and hear spirit sounds as well as feel the spirits pass by me.

I was still a little suspicious. I wondered about all of the windows being covered and asked the women how they knew that the shaman wasn't performing conjuring tricks and fooling them into thinking that something spiritual was happening during the ceremony. They told me that so much activity takes place that if there were any people moving around they would trip over chairs, possibly impale themselves on flagsticks, and in general find it very difficult to "see" in the dark. She was convinced that Doug would bring spirits into the room.

By that time we were all assembled, or at least I thought we were. We sat and chatted with each other. As we sat there I asked what we were waiting for. They told me that the "singer" hadn't shown up yet. I wondered who or what the "singer" was. As I pondered this, Doug proceeded to open a brown suitcase he had carried with him into the room. It was quite small, so I assumed that it contained a few artifacts needed for the ceremony. I was mistaken. In the case was more than I expected it could hold. As he unloaded it, placing the various objects on the floor, I had the impression that I was watching a magician performing an ancient feat of magic. You know the kind of trick where the magician pulls an endless number of objects, which couldn't possibly fit inside, from a box on the floor.

When he had finished, the living room floor had been transformed into an altar-stage called a *Hocoka*, containing all of the ritual accouterments that he would need to perform the ceremony. The first thing he took from the case was a rug that he carefully placed on the floor. The rug was darkly colored, appearing quite black, and quite large – at least seven by ten feet. He then took a peace pipe from the case. It had a long stem and its bowl was made from red pipestone. It was roughly carved in the shape of a figure that I could not discern. He also pulled four small flags in solid colors of red, blue, yellow, and white from the case. He attached the flags to four sticks, each about three feet in length. Each color represented a spiritual force from a different direction. White represented the south, Red, the North, Yellow, the East, and Blue, the West. Usually black is used instead of blue.

Later, one of the women brought in four coffee cans filled halfway with dirt. Doug placed each of the miniature "flagpoles" in a separate can and placed the cans at the four corners of the dark carpet, marking off the appropriate directions of space. He also placed some eagle feathers on the rug toward the end facing the chairs in the middle line of the three-sided square.

As he continued to prepare the altar, the "singer" appeared in the doorway. His name was Marvin Red Elk. I was struck by his appearance. He was a young full-blooded Oglala Sioux with long black hair tied in the back in a ponytail. His skin was richly reddish brown, and his quite handsome face was strikingly marked by slanting but full brown eyes. He carried a large flat drum with him, at least eighteen inches to two feet in diameter, and a striker to play the drum.

With the arrival of Marvin, Doug took off his shirt and his shoes and socks. He was surprisingly fit for a man who smoked like a chimney and apparently drank booze. But, as I mentioned, the booze impression was incorrect, as were most of my early impressions of him. Nevertheless, he was nearly seventy years old. I noticed that he had many wounds on his chest, mainly centered around his breasts. These were wounds given to him in the traditional Plains Indian ceremony known as the "sun dance." He also had several scars on his arms. These were from skin offerings.

He then put two large rattles on the rug. They were covered in buffalo hide. Inside the gourds were many small stones or seeds and dried pieces of his own skin. Doug then told me that no rings could be worn during the ceremony, and certainly no silver. So everyone was asked to remove any rings or silver from the hands or neck. Then a string of tiny purses, looking like small tea bags, containing tobacco and called *canli wapahte*, were strung out like popcorn strands at Christmas from flag to flag, making the area look like a small boxing ring.

When all this was in place, the closed-off area was regarded as a re-creation of the universe as seen by the Oglala Indians. The space was thus transformed from a profane or everyday state into a sacred model of the universe.

Just as we were ready to begin the ceremony, Doug, standing in the middle of the rug, turned to me and surprisingly began to joke with me. He then said, "You're going to get scared. But it is very important that you offer a prayer for Paul and me." I felt quite honored that he thought that my prayers were important. As he stood there preparing for the event I suddenly realized – with total conviction, this time – that Doug was not a drunken Indian but a powerful shaman and that all of the early experiences I had with him were just preparations and illusions to throw me off guard, to see if I was worthy enough to engage in what was about to come.

Then the lights in the room were turned out. He asked if anyone could see any light. I noticed that some light was coming in from the window near me. Doug asked me to adjust the blanket over the window. I did. He also asked anyone in the room who was wearing glasses to remove them. I removed mine. Then Marvin began chanting and playing the drum. His voice resonated throughout the room. Later on I found out that Marvin was an accomplished artist as well as a ceremonial singer. I was quite spellbound by the song he sang and felt as if I were floating.

As I sat there in the dark, I suddenly saw flashes of light coming from different places in the room. At first I suspected that Doug was striking a pocket cigarette lighter, however, I didn't hear any sound associated with these flashes. The light also didn't appear to be produced by a flashlight, either. The color of the lights was a greenish blue. The lights appeared to be like the glows from large fireflies. Then I heard the flutter of wings. The spirits had come into the room.

Later I found out that these apparitions were signals of the spirits that were summoned by Doug to help in the complete healing of Paul. The

Oglala shaman operates differently than some shamans who go on a journey to the spirit world to diagnose and heal the sick. Instead the Oglala shamans call the spirits, powers from the past, into the present, and their manifestation is signaled by the flashing lights and eagle wings beating.

The Yuwipi shaman is an intermediary between the supernatural and the common people, the dead and the living, the past and the present. Through this mediation the present world is placed in contact with "all of our relations."

The term "all my relations," *Mitak' oyas'in*, is very important. It is recited after each person has said his prayer in the ceremony.

Doug then began reciting a prayer to the six spiritual directions. Later I found out that Marvin had sung this prayer in his song. Loosely translated it goes:

Friend, I will send a voice, so hear me.
Friend, I will send a voice, so hear me.
Friend, I will send a voice, so hear me.
Friend, I will send a voice, so hear me.

In the West I call a black stone friend.
Friend, I will send a voice, so hear me.
Friend, I will send a voice, so hear me.

In the North I call a red stone friend.
Friend, I will send a voice, so hear me.
Friend, I will send a voice, so hear me.

In the East I call a yellow stone friend.
Friend, I will send a voice, so hear me.
Friend, I will send a voice, so hear me.

In the South I call a white stone friend.
Friend, I will send a voice, so hear me.
Friend, I will send a voice, so hear me.

On earth, I will call a spider friend.
Friend, I will send a voice, so hear me.
Friend, I will send a voice, so hear me.

Above, I will call a spotted eagle friend.
Friend, I will send a voice, so hear me.
Friend, I will send a voice, so hear me.

This song is considered to be the most powerful chant in the ceremony because it si directed to the entire universe. It reminded me of the three mutually perpendicular directions of space, and the dimension of time. By bringing the spirits through the past, the dimension of time is brought in, so the whole four-dimensional space-time continuum is evoked in the ceremony.

After the song and the prayer by Doug, I heard violent shakings of the rattles. I nearly jumped out of my chair when suddenly one of the rattles struck the floor between my legs. I was quite shaken. I was also amazed when I realized that when the gourd struck the ground it glowed the same brilliant blue-green color as the "fireflies: I had seen earlier.

After thinking about it, I realized that the color was similar to that produced by a phosphorescent material. However, I had never seen a material phosphoresce in the manner when it was struck against another object. Perhaps it was some form of static electrical discharge. On a dry night, if you rub the folds of a nylon or other synthetic fabric blanket together you can produce sparks of color that are similar to what I saw. However, this explanation doesn't quite work for the flashes I saw, because the sparks are always accompanied by the sounds of the sparks. These colors flashed silently.

The whole ceremony continued in this manner. There were songs, chants, and prayers by Doug and the continual surprises of flashing lights and eagle wings. Quite often the flashes and wingbeats were only inches from my face and body, and each time it happened, I was startled. After about an hour, the room grew silent. Doug asked each person in the room to offer a prayer. Although I was the only white person in the room, not all of the Sioux present spoke the Sioux language. But each one offered a prayer.

It was then that I realized how seriously these people took the experience. I heard many different kinds of prayer. Some wished for better health. Others wanted to have their personal relationships improve. A few were bothered by spirits and asked if other spirits would come into their homes and clean out the bad spirits.

I was moved by the humble and open spirits of my new friends, and I felt as if I were a part of their family. A kind of relationship or feeling of relatedness took place in the room. I remember another ceremony like it. I once attended a Narcotics-Alcoholics Anonymous meeting with my son, Michael, and felt a similar presence of spiritual force when each person "confessed" and told honestly about his life and problems with drug abuse.

When my turn came, I offered a prayer. I first prayed for Doug and Paul's safe journey to Canada, as I was instructed to. I thanked "all my relations" present in the room for inviting me to partake in the experience. I then offered a prayer for better understanding and more felt love between the many peoples of the world. After each prayer, the ensemble would say "Ho," signifying the acceptance of me and my prayer. I felt that my prayer was moving to them and I believed that they took what I said to heart.

Then the ceremony was officially ended, and the lights were turned on. I then thought over the experience and realized that all of us were still seated in our chairs, and yet during the darkness, I had felt as if the room was full of moving people. With the room lights on I then looked at the altar. Everything that was laid out was completely scattered about. Some of the cans had dirt spilled out around them, and everything was in disarray.

I was astonished when I looked up at Doug. He was standing in the middle of the altar space with blood dripping form a cut just under his right eye.

Doug then quietly said to one of the women who had helped him set up the room, "You forgot to include the raw beef liver in the altar. The spirits were angry at this." He didn't offer any reason for his bleeding. But I surmised that it was a mark from the spirits because he forgot to include the liver in the ceremony.

Then Doug turned to me. He began to kid me again in a good-natured manner. He wanted to know if I was very frightened during the ceremony. I got the feeling that it was better for me to tell him the truth and say how frightened I was. That gave him a good laugh. I told him that I was very frightened and that, when the rattle banged on the floor between my legs, I nearly jumped out of my chair. He was laughing and nearly rolling on the floor. I told him that if that gourd came any closer to me, I would have jumped out of the window. He howled with laughter. He then proceeded to gather up all of the materials he had placed on the floor and put them back into his small suitcase.

Paul got up from his chair and went into the kitchen. Several deep cooking pots were placed in the middle of the floor. Each contained a typical Sioux food. One had a stew in it. Another had a jam made from chokecherries. Fried bread was offered, which tasted very much like sopapillas served in New Mexico. Jell-O was offered and Kool-Aid or coffee was served. Everything was quite tasty, and I enjoyed myself. I was surprised at how hungry I was.

As we were sitting around digesting our food, I noticed that Doug had eaten very little. Apparently he was used to fasting and felt little hunger. I then mentioned to everyone that first they frighten me and then they fatten me up. Doug laughed at that, and all of the people there joined in, in good spirit. I told him that even though the lights were now on, I still felt the presence of the spirits. Doug nodded his head in acknowledgement and enjoyed my spontaneous offering of humor and my playing the part of the fool.

Later each of them told me that he or she had been frightened the first time when going through such a ceremony. My lack of bravado was refreshing to them. Then, as it was now quite late, I went up to each person shook his or her hand, and said thanks for having me. I said good-bye and walked outside to get to my car. Doug then said, "Be careful when you drive. Watch out for playful spirits."

Doug and Paul then followed me out. As we stood in the moonlight, Doug said that when he got back from Canada, he would take me up to a mountain for a vision quest, if I wanted it. I didn't feel very keen about the idea, because I was afraid that his Heyokah spirit would make me too upset. Perhaps I was being a "chicken." Perhaps I was being prudent. He would be to me as Don Juan was to Carlos Castañeda. He would be perhaps my "petty tyrant." I remembered how he had fooled me throughout the day, at first appearing as a drunken Indian, somewhat incoherent, and then as a powerful shaman fully in control of his physical and spiritual faculties. When I first met him, he appeared old and shrunken. When he performed the ceremony, he appeared tall and youthful.

I was about to get in my car when Doug approached me again and said, "Now when you drive home, remember to look straight ahead." He then turned away and went to a vacant space on the land, bent over at the waist and threw up what little he had consumed. I was again reminded of the drunken Indian image. Was he just sick with booze? I still doubted.

After seeing that Doug was okay, I just said good-bye and got into my car, little suspecting (although I was warned) that my journey into the spirit world was not over yet. I drove carefully along the dirt road leading out to the highway threading through the reservation. I remembered to turn right to get back to the medical compound where I was staying in Pine Ridge.

I was driving along feeing quite content when I suddenly realized that I was driving in the wrong direction. I must have driven around ten miles when I felt this. I turned around and proceeded back, bemoaning that it was late and that I would have to drive at least another twenty of so miles before I would get home. I was getting quite tired.

After driving for around fifteen miles I again had the feeling I was going in the wrong direction. I was totally confused. So I turned around once again and headed back in the same direction I had originally taken when I reached the highway. Finally, after driving about an hour, a trip that should have taken me no more than fifteen minutes, I managed to make my way back to Pine Ridge and my apartment on the compound. The jokester-shaman was still playing with me.

I left the next day for New Mexico. I had finally been exposed to a Native American shamanic ritual. It was not the last I was to experience.

THE ALCOVE OF DEATH

BILL PLOTKIN

IN THE WILD ORCHARD, SOUL-ROOTED INDIVIDUATION, INCLUDING integration of the four dimensions of the Self, is often catalyzed or amplified by numinous experiences. For me more than once, this has happened through encounters with Death.

Sometimes we're granted the chance to meet with Death as a perceptible presence in addition to confronting the inevitability of our own mortality. The first time I spoke directly and tangibly to Death was in a redrock canyon in southern Utah not long after entering the Wild Orchard.

Some years earlier, Steve Zeller and I took our first hike down Grotto Canyon to look for basecamps for future vision fast groups. We came to the mouth of one of its tributaries and decided to have a look. A minute up the side canyon, Steve sat down without explanation and said he'd wait there. He waved me on with an odd smile. As I continued, the chasm began to feel a bit creepy, but nothing I could identify specifically. A sense of foreboding. Deciding it didn't feel so good up there, I turned back and told Steve what happened. He said, "No kidding. There was no way I was going up there." We didn't speak about it further.

A few years later, another friend, Dave, returned from a solo hike in Grotto Canyon. He told me he ventured into a side canyon and up a steep south-facing slope to a giant alcove in the upper wall. He said he'd felt strongly pulled by something. He peered into the dark interior of the alcove. When his eyes adjusted, he recoiled. He wouldn't tell me exactly what he saw but said, with wide eyes, that his name for that place was Death Alcove. He did not go in.

I found the topographic map of Grotto and asked Dave to identify the alcove's location. He pointed to the north wall of the same side canyon that Steve and I had entered.

Within a year, Judy, another friend (who does not know Dave) took a winter hike down Grotto Canyon with her dog, Lucky. She said there was one place in particular that really got her attention. It had scared her — no, terrified her. It was an alcove high on the wall of one of the many side canyons. The hair on the back of my neck stirred. I asked her what was frightening about it. She said there was something odd on the back wall but emphasized that it was really the whole feeling of the place. Lucky wouldn't go any nearer the alcove and barked wildly when Judy did. Judy, standing at the alcove's mouth, soon grew frightened and she and Lucky fled. She told me that she came to think of that place as "the Alcove of Death." I pulled out my topo. Same place.

Two years later, in May, I was in the lower end of Grotto Canyon leading an eight-day soulcraft program. There were twelve of us. We had not planned to be in that canyon that week, but my intended destination, a place I call the Cemetery, was unreachable that spring due to heavy winter snows still blocking the access road. I had planned a group exercise in the Cemetery that involved a ritual encounter with Death. I told the group my aborted plans. They wanted to enact the ceremony anyway and asked if there wasn't an appropriate location in Grotto? I said no, it needed to be done in the Cemetery. They insisted I must know a spot that would work.

Then I remembered the Alcove. I told them I knew of a place that might work but that it was too far and I had never actually been there and, for that matter, I wasn't sure I could even find it. Besides, it would take half a day to hike that far up the main canyon and another half to return by nightfall. To my chagrin, they all wanted to go and wouldn't hear otherwise.

The real reason I didn't want to go was because of what I had promised myself I would do in the Cemetery ceremony. For several months, I had been feeling a need to commit myself more fully to my soul work. Any of my friends, if asked, would have said that that was ludicrous, but on some level I really believed I was still holding back. So it came to me that the thing to do was to return to the Cemetery — a place where the presence of Death was, for me, quite palpable — and to make a sacred vow in Death's presence. Given how I intended to frame that vow, the prospect of actually doing it was rather intimidating.

As soon as I remembered the Alcove of Death, I realized it would be a location at least as fitting as the Cemetery. Maybe more so.

The next day we arose before dawn, packed for a full day, and headed upstream. I grew more anxious by the step. After five tiring hours, we reached the mouth of the side canyon. Looking high on its north wall, I immediately saw the alcove with its dark entrance yawning into the bright day. There were also two smaller alcoves on the same wall further to the east, lower and closer to where we stood. I turned around to the man behind me, a very intuitive and compassionate person. I pointed to the alcove furthest to the east, and said, unconvincingly, that that must be our destination. Michael laughed, put his arm around me, and said he knew I knew otherwise and that there was no way of getting out of this.

Resigned, I told the group that we'd hike up the slope until we found the right spot to prepare ourselves, a place where we'd ask each person two very poignant and difficult questions. When the ceremony had come to me several weeks earlier, I only knew that this staging area would be known as the Place of the Questions. There we would enact a ceremonial group-consensus process to determine who was and who was not psychologically prepared to enter the alcove — based upon each person's answers to the two questions. Only those who received unanimous consent would go the rest of the way, and they would go alone, one at a time.

Ascending the narrow chasm of stream-polished red sandstone, we climbed steeply, threading our way through a massive tumble of boulders on petrified sand dunes until we came to the base of a house-sized rock. Climbing left around the shadowed base and then to the top of the rock, we found that it had a flat roof just large enough for the twelve of us to gather in a circle. Only a few feet from where we stood, in the direction of the alcove high above, was a giant yucca — a "century plant" that sends up a twelve-foot stalk of blossoms. This particular yucca stalk had grown and then dried into the exact shape of a giant question mark. With a wry smile, I remarked that we had apparently found the place to ask the questions.

It was mid-day, the sky was flawlessly blue, and it was hot on that jumbled slope of baking rocks. When I was granted permission to go, I pulled off my T-shirt and scrambled full speed, hands and feet, up the incline as the others drummed below. The aerobic effort briefly kept my fear in check. My primary objective was to look Death in the eye — if he was really there — and make a solemn declaration of my soul work, and ask him to take my life anytime my commitment should falter.

Reaching the alcove, I stopped, heart beating wildly and feeling very small on the edge of such an immense space. The shadowed cavern was about 100 feet deep and at least that high and twice as wide at its mouth. An undisturbed slope of pure tan sand ran steeply up from my feet toward the back wall. A single large clump of sacred datura, whose large while flowers are sometimes used as a hallucinogen and can be lethal, once grew in the center of the sand slope, but it was long dead, its gray branches now a mass of desiccated bones two feet high. There were no other signs of previous life or habitation in this place.

Then I saw, on the back wall, a thin, ten-foot tall humanoid figure in high-relief, apparently formed from minerals leaching from water seeps in the soft sandstone. Dressed in a long emerald, gold, and black flowing robe, he gazed down at me with hollow eyes and a terrible aura of omniscience. Involuntarily I dropped to my knees in the sand. If I were really going to do it, this was the moment. Trembling, breathless, I began to describe my soul work, my commitment to it, and my request that he be my most fierce ally by holding my life as surety for my vow.

As I spoke, Death nodded, but with what seemed like an air of impatience and indifference, perhaps some amusement. Uncertain, I kept speaking. He began pointing to his left without ever shifting his gaze from me. When I finished, he said, "You can make whatever promises you want, but they're of no interest to me until you make a commitment to her." He gestured again to his left.

Only then did I see her, a similarly robed figure, not quite as tall, standing next to him, his left arm embracing her shoulders. Dumbfounded, I looked back at him and he said, "This is my wife, Joy."

In that moment, my understanding of Death and of my own life shattered. It was as if a cathedral had crumbled around me and I stood in billowing dust. This was the last thing I could have imagined hearing from Death. Abruptly, the old symbols were gone, there were no scriptures to consult, no questions to ask, and the only possible actions meaningless.

"She is as much a presence in eternity as me," Death continued. "You have some awareness of mortality and a beginning relationship with me, but you have little affiliation with Joy. Your soul work will not progress further until you surrender to her. Don't come back until you have."

As he spoke, my perceptual experience of the alcove was shifting radically. Upon arrival, it felt like I had imagined it would — a foreboding place that only heroes or fools would visit. Now it emanated a sweet aura, a sanctified glow something like I'd expect of a honeymoon cottage. The Alcove now felt more like a marital abode for Death and Joy, a playground for their eternal romance.

Overwhelmed and disoriented, I turned and staggered slowly down the slope. I felt both ruined and gifted by an encounter I would not have known how to imagine. On that day, I began my apprenticeship to Joy — a teacher who stands partnered with Death.

An embrace of joy had indeed not been my strong point. I tend to be overly earnest. I had expected Death to help me become even more assiduous, but, in fact, he directed me toward what I now see was my least developed faculty — light-heartedness, playfulness, simplicity, and my capacity to surrender to joy. These things are not just needed to round out my personality and humanity; they're also essential ingredients for growing deeper into my soul work.

Since that visit to the Alcove of Death, I have come to think of that place as the Alcove of Love, a celebration of the alchemy between Death and Joy who, joined, exist as Love. A dark and foreboding place becomes a doorway to our true home. We are irrevocably altered by walking, ceremonially, toward what we most fear.

Dance as Life: Completing the Circle

Christauria Welland

For as long as I can remember, I have been a dancer. Dance flows out of the core of my being, expressing deep emotions, spiritual peace, and the essence of my thoughts. When asked to draw a person by a psychologist years ago, I drew a young woman in a flowing dress, dancing joyfully. Although that year was the lowest point of my life and I was undergoing a pitch-black depression, somewhere, deep in my heart, *I* was still there, not yet lost, not yet beyond hope.

Dance is not only art. Dance is often sacred ritual, especially outside of Western circles. In the West, many traditions and mind-body expressions of the interior person have been lost to daily practice. We are cut off from our bodies in so many ways. The journey of human existence is a long road towards integration of the sacred and the secular, the spiritual and the sensual, the emotional and the intellectual. Our bodies are an integral part of this quest for union. Saints of every stripe have attempted to slough off the body prematurely, undergoing astounding penances so as to reach their spiritual goal. On the other hand, in the contemporary West and increasingly in other regions, we indulge and pamper our bodies to such a degree that we have misplaced the ability to live on any other plane. Somewhere between these two extremes lies the middle path, trodden by a multitude of holy people through the ages - the path of balance and love for the Divine, for self, and for neighbor.

In ritual we utilize the visible to signify and enact the invisible thought,

199

belief, spiritual reality. We use music, sacred objects, the elements, sacred actions, movements, and often, dance. The universality of ritual suggests that it is an integral part of human development, perhaps demonstrating that we have a profound need to act together, to create meaningful bonds, and to outwardly signify events or beliefs of perennial value that we do not wish to lose or forget. Holding and celebrating these essential values and beliefs in common ensures their survival.

Dance as a sacred ritual and integral part of religious expression has been present in all religions at some point. The sacred dances of the early Christians in Europe were probably linked to the influence of their Jewish heritage, and have long been lost to time (Kirk, 1983). Attempts to revive sacred dance in a Christian context have been peripheral to modern liturgical renewal in the West. Jews, however, still dance as part of their wedding ceremony. Rumi and the Mevlevi dervishes of the Sufi tradition used dance as an avenue to enlightenment.

Dance, when you're broken open.
Dance, if you've torn the bandage off.
Dance in the middle of the fighting.
Dance in your blood.
Dance, when you're perfectly free

(tr Barks, 2003, p. 281).

For many tribal peoples in Africa and India, ritual and tradition without communal dance is unthinkable. Many Christian churches in these regions incorporate the deeply felt need for physical expression through dance and music into sacred rituals that make their celebrations profoundly different from those in Western churches. In the traditions of the Catholic Yaqui and Rarámuri (Tarahumara) peoples of northern Mexico, sacred dance is intimately linked to survival through the planting and hunting rituals that include community and individual dance, sacramentalizing the sacrifice of the deer or the growth of the sacred corn. Being present at some of these sacred rituals -- in the dead of a cold spring night while bonfires roar and homemade beer flows freely – have been some of the most exhilarating moments of my life. The unity and fellowship evoked in sacred communal dance cannot be duplicated in any other way.

Powwows that bring together the sacred dancing rituals of the native peoples of the Americas are rich opportunities to experience oneself as part of the rhythm of the universe and the human family at a level that pounds in unison with your heartbeat. The sacred Deer Dance of the Yaquis transcends the limits between human and animal and transforms the hunt into a participation in the mystery of life itself. Swaying from side to side, Aztec dancers stomp and swirl to the sound of the drums, with walnut shells rattling and feather headdresses towering overhead -- in front of a Catholic altar after the celebration of the Mass on a Mexican feast day. These are moments to feel your humanity, to stomp into the ground the existential loneliness and emptiness that plague us.

I began the formal study of classical ballet when I was 10 years old, which seemed an impossibly long wait to me. When I was 13, I added modern dance to my studies. Looking back, I realize how being engrossed in this art throughout my adolescence was my salvation from a multitude of dangers and potential disasters. My parents were in the throes of a divorce and preoccupied with their own struggles. It was the sixties, and drugs were everywhere, upheaval was everywhere. Everything was called into question. A magnificent time to be alive, a time of excitement, and yes, confusion. I didn't have the answers, but I was determined to find my own way. Dance kept me centered, grounded, focused, with the experience of mastery that built up my self-concept in an uncertain world and an uncertain family. Dance was the place where my natural expressiveness and deep passions could find their voice.

Classical ballet is a dance form that was created to entertain the elite of Europe. As such, ballet has never had roots in a ritual, spiritual significance. As challenging and satisfying as it is to master impossible leg extensions, complex pirouettes *en pointe*, and great leaps through the ether to land gracefully and effortlessly in the arms of your partner, it is also representative of the divorce from the earth, from nature, that characterizes much of Western culture. Many ballet positions go against the natural form of the body: the turnout of the legs and feet; standing and turning on the tiny circumference of the *pointe* shoe, two sizes smaller than your feet; squashing your toes into spaces that stunt and deform their growth. In spite of this, I had my heart set on a dance career, and with the blessing of my teachers and the economic support of my parents, I headed to Paris in 1969, just in time to catch the tail end of the great student demonstrations of the sixties. I had seen the *Ballet du XXe Siècle (Ballet of the 20th Century)* of Maurice Béjart in Montreal, and I knew that this was the company I wanted to join. His principal dance teacher, a graceful and forceful Russian named Tatiana Grantzeva, had her studio in Montmartre in Paris. Béjart's choreography incorporated spiritual themes like the *Dark Night of the Soul* by St. John of the Cross, and tales of Eastern spirituality and mysticism. There was meaning in his art, not just technique, form, virtuosity, and expression. My soul longed for meaning; technique was no longer enough.

In one of those coincidences in life that change the course of everything and make you wonder if coincidences really exist, I came upon my first sight of the Indian classical dance Bharata Natyam in Paris, while I was looking for my weekly modern dance class. I was transfixed by the sight and the movement of the beautiful and tranquil Amala Devi, with her long black braid and orange sari, showing some simple dance moves to two French girls. Spellbound, I knew in an instant that this was what I had to do. Ever the dramatist and demonstrating my innate love of ritual, I bid Madame Grantzeva farewell and carefully placed my *pointe* shoes in the garbage bin outside her studio. It was my nineteenth birthday, and I had broken with Western dance.

My Bharata Natyam classes began the next week, and within months I had returned to Ottawa and obtained a scholarship from the Indian Council for Cultural Relations to study Bharata Natyam in India. Amala encouraged me to live in Bangalore, and to study under the gurus U.S. Krishna Rao and his wife U. K. Chandrabhaga Devi (Chandamma), not only because of their renown as dancers and teachers, but also because of their fluency in English, experience with Western culture, and Bangalore's forgiving, relatively temperate climate, compared with other centers of the art in South India.

My journey to India began in January 1971, while I was still 19. It was a transformative spiritual quest, a stripping down to essentials, and a radical acceptance of interdependence on the Divine, the goodness of others, and the choice to risk everything to obtain a goal. As for all who are on pilgrimage, "the journey is inward and outward at the same time" (Zaleski & Kaufman, 1997, p. 138). Wherever I went, traveling overland to India, I practiced yoga and Bharata Natyam. Dance was bringing order into my personal and familial chaos, structuring my inner life as it structured my body and its place in space, in the universe. When the body moves and expresses itself, knowing is on a deeper, more integrated level. Understanding moves beyond the confines of linear thought.

I arrived in Bangalore in April 1971. Krishna Rao was a man in his early sixties, his wife ten years younger. My new gurus' kindness and warmth enveloped me like parental love from the moment I arrived in India. Sure of himself and of his goals as a master and teacher of dance, Krishna Rao started me on a daily regimen of private lessons that lasted 3 to 4 hours, beginning in the cool of the morning. Since Bharata Natyam is an ancient tradition that has been passed on for centuries, there was a great deal to learn about every aspect of the art: the expression of emotions, the multitude of *mudras* (hand movements), sometimes signifying the story line and sometimes perfecting the pure movement of the dance. The dances required me to learn the stories of Hindu mythology, and Krishna Rao quickly understood my spiritual longings. He sat with me and effortlessly explained the deeper spiritual meaning of the stories, as expressions of the soul yearning for or attaining union with the Divine. Bharata Natyam is very much a *bhakti* (devotional) form of Hindu expression. Chandamma took me to temple rituals and prayers, where I was swept into the current of Hindu devotion to the gods and goddesses. Although I never became a Hindu, I developed a deep respect and intuitive grasp of Indian yearning for divine unity. India became the womb of my spiritual rebirth.

During this memorable 18-month period, I was also in the midst of an intense search to decide to which religion to give my heart and mind. Over time it became clear to me that my path lay with the Catholic faith, on account of the mystical teachings of the saints and the astounding sacred experience that is the Mass. Simultaneously, I had volunteered for a month in the refugee camps of West Bengal, since the war in what is now Bangla Desh was raging, and 10 million people had fled the violence. It became increasingly clear to me that I must dedicate my life to the service of the poor and destitute. Being a religious sister seemed the best way to go about this, for the work of Catholic sisters in India was a great light illuminating those who lived in darkness and suffering on the fringes of society. I took instructions from the Apostolic Carmelite sisters in Bangalore and began to volunteer with the Missionaries of Charity. By November of 1971, I had met with Mother Teresa in Calcutta and had been invited to enter the Sisters. Standing in an empty lot near my home in Bangalore on the night of December 7, I looked up at the dark sky scattered with stars and told God that I would give up dance to serve him with my whole heart, but that I would have to dance forever in heaven. To this day, I have never made a sacrifice that cost me more.

When I entered the Missionaries of Charity in Calcutta, at the age of 21, my gurus were sad and disappointed, and assured me that I was making a huge mistake. My family and friends were in disbelief. But I have never regretted that decision, whatever its cost.

Within 2 years, I had injured my back to such a degree that surgeries were necessary, and a spinal fusion assured that I would never again be a dancer on this earth. The work was intense and eventually dried up the emotional current of the new convert, as is to be expected in the spiritual life. I was high and dry, with only my faith in Christ and the tenacious belief that my life was making a difference in the lives of the poorest of the poor. Over the next 19 years, chronic pain and emotional and physical trauma took a deep toll. Surrounded by slums and the grinding poverty and injustice that strains anyone's ability to keep believing and hoping in God and in goodness, I found myself weeping, longing to simply be able to admire and touch a flower, or anything beautiful. Eventually, my physical and emotional health broke down completely. Once I had taken medical leave with the Benedictine sisters in San Diego, I knew that going back would mean a certain return to the state I was in. I had to move forward to survive.

Sixteen years passed. I made San Diego my home, married and completed a doctoral degree in clinical psychology. I spent many hours in therapy with understanding people who supported me in the drastic changes in my life and in the painful process of healing. The pieces of my body, mind, heart, and soul began to come back together. I worked as I always had, with the neediest people around me, the ones that no one seemed to remember or take account of. Back problems continued to keep me from dance.

In 2006, 35 years after I left India, I contacted old friends in South India, and my husband and I embarked on a journey to my spiritual home. In the gentle heat and pouring rain of the November monsoon, we toured Tamil Nadu, visiting some of the most important and ancient centers of Bharata Natyam in the state. In the sacred city of Kanchipuram, we pilgrimaged to the shrine of Kamakshi Amman, one of three surviving temples dedicated to Shakti, the female cosmic energy, and the place where Kamakshi, or Parvati (Shiva's consort) is worshipped. Although the inner sanctum is off bounds to non-Hindus, we received a blessing from the trunk of one of the temple elephants, and were able to circumambulate the shrine as evening fell on the brightly illuminated golden dome of the sanctuary. This is the temple where the brilliant Balasaraswati, a legendary dancer of Bharata Natyam whose artistry and spiritual dedication to dance was the apex of the revival of the art in the 20th century, offered her first performance (*aranget-ram*) to the goddess at the age of nine. I saw Balasaraswati in Bangalore in 1971; my gurus considered a glimpse of her artistic achievement essential to my training. When you see a momentary facial expression or a flick of the finger move the universe, you know you are in the presence of genius. Balasaraswati did not dance with her whole body that night, for reasons I do not know. However, just to see her cross-legged on her little platform, moving only her upper body, was to be transported into the presence of Shakti in all her refulgent purity and energy.

On this trip, we boarded the early morning train to reach Tiruchi-rapalli and then a taxi to Shantivanam Ashram, a Catholic monastery, where I lived for several months in 1972, delving deeper into Catholic teaching, spirituality, and prayer with Bede Griffiths and the monks. The chapel where I used to dance before the altar during the presentation of gifts at the Mass had been enlarged, but was otherwise the same, with its darkened sanctuary where the Eucharist resides. I prostrated myself and kissed the mat, giving thanks for the opportunity to return to sacred ground. That night, when communal prayers were over and everyone had gone, I danced to the Lord before that altar again. Sharing in the silent life of the monastery for a few days was balm, and a quiet cycling back to a time of great upheaval and transformation in my life. Shifts in my spirit that I did not even know were wanting fell tranquilly into place. The circle was closing and the grief of loss, of lost parts of myself, was assuaged.

We drove through a torrential downpour during the entire journey to Madurai, a city with a history that stretches back over 2000 years. In the careening vehicle, I prepared myself to set foot in the great temple of Meenakshi (another manifestation of Parvati, Shiva's consort), by practicing the Sanskrit songs my guru taught me in 1971. At Meenakshi's shrine, one of the most sacred of India's temples, Bharata Natyam was performed for centuries to honor the deities. Materializing from a cloud of sandalwood incense, dark and heavily sculpted pillared hallways filled with vendors and copious garlands of flowers and offerings to the goddess lead to the gigantic courtyard. There the 150-foot high *gopuras* -- insanely bright, painted towers encrusted with thousands of scenes from Hindu mythology -- stand guard around the Golden Lotus Tank, where worshippers bathe ritually before entering the twin sanctums of Meenakshi and Shiva. Since we could not enter there, our guide took us to the Ayirakkal Mandapa, the Hall of a Thousand Pillars, where an enormous statue of Shiva Nataraj draped with silk garlands adorns a platform in the inmost reaches of the hall. Unusually for a temple where thousands of pilgrims visit daily, there were no other visitors when we entered.

Grasping the unexpected opportunity without a second's thought, I began the *namaskaram*, the ritual salutation to the deity that consecrates the whole of the dancer, body, mind and spirit, to God and the performance of the sacred dance. Accompanying myself in song, I performed *Deva Payat*, a *sloka* (verse) taken from the ancient Sanskrit writings of the Hindu sages. My technique was shaky, and I forgot some of the choreography my master had so carefully taught me, but I completed it with an exaltation I have rarely felt. When I finished, a small group of about 50 students that had gathered around unbeknownst to me burst into applause.

My dance was an act of worship to the mighty Lord, an offering of my whole life, past, present, and future, to the One who holds our fortunes and our hopes in all-powerful hands. Exaltation flowed from surrender, from total gift, from acceptance of reality in the moment, in the absence of image, thought, or words. Worship, true and profound joy, forgetfulness of self –- these are my attempts to describe the ineffable state that lies beyond verbal conception.

Inside my soul, something clicked into place. The sacrifice of my life as a dancer was somehow complete. The homage before Shiva, lord of the dance and of creation, had removed the thorn of loss and replaced it with the original sense I once had of knowing and valuing my place in the sacred dance of creation. My heart stopped bleeding and a new integration blossomed.

Dance, if you've torn the bandage off... Dance, when you're perfectly free.

Beyond the immediate enthrallment of dancing in that sacred hall, over the next week it was as if I had rediscovered my deepest, truest being without any conscious effort or reflection. Body and soul were united once again. The circle was closed, with just a little space for Spirit to get through on another day, at another time, when least expected.

The relative quiet of this area can be attributed to the small entrance fee, since there is also an art museum within the hall.

References

Barks, C. (2003). Rumi: The book of love: Poems of love and longing. HarperCollins: San Francisco.

Kardong, T.G. (1996). Benedict's Rule: A Translation and Commentary. St Johns, MN: Liturgical Press.

Kirk, M.A. (1983). Dancing with creation: Mexican and Native American dance in Christian worship and education. Saratoga, CA: Resource Publications.

Zaleski. P. & Kaufman, P. (1997). Gifts of the Spirit: Living the Wisdom of the Great Religious Traditions. HarperCollins: San Francisco.

RITUAL AS CONVEYANCE: THE BEAR

JEANNIE BECK

THE FIRST FORMAL RITUAL I WAS EVER INVOLVED IN WAS A NATIVE American sweat, held at a nearby reservation several years ago. The leader was an Indian man from the Los Coyotes Reservation, in San Diego County. I'd met Merley some twenty-five years past, when we were both teenagers drinking beer at a party. After choosing sobriety, I'd heard he'd gone on to do a lot of healing work for people with substance abuse problems in the surrounding communities. Through mutual acquaintances, I learned he was holding sweats out on the reservation for anyone who felt the need. I'd had it in mind for years to attend a sweat but hadn't made the connection. Well, I sort of knew this guy, and here it was not too far from home. This was my easy opportunity. As it turned out, there was nothing easy about it.

It involved more than a physical sort of sweating. Early on I viewed my experience as an exercise in will, and then it became a practice of surrendering that will. In the end I saw it as neither gaining nor losing control, but something interactive, like driving. Ultimately, I came to realize the value of ritual lay in the offering of a vehicle. It has the potential to move you to places you might have reached more slowly, or perhaps not at all, if left to your own devices. The ritual itself has a distinct persona that can carry you beyond the place you might have stopped without it. In the case of a sweat you are actively involved, like it or not, and to participate requires extreme discomfort. You are forced to levels of experience previously unknown. Beyond endurance, a new awareness, a transformation of consciousness. is possible. I think the appeal of ritual is its enduring form, ripe with potential should you choose to enter it again. It has the power, if only temporarily, to alter and expand your perceptions.

I arrived about sunset as several men were chopping logs and stoking a blazing fire. There were the hippie whites, the Indians, the successful new-agers, and a few stray unclassifieds. I was the one unprepared, unversed. Perhaps people wondered if I'd merely gotten lost and stumbled in, and what the hell, I guess I'll check it out. I only admit to the ravings of my mind to show you how self-conscious and out of place I felt. I hadn't fasted, wasn't dressed right, and didn't really know anybody. What if I collapsed or did something embarrassing?

A group of people was seated on a large blanket mindfully tying strings to brightly colored bits of cloth filled with tobacco. These were prayers we were fashioning, but I must confess, my main prayer was that no one would notice that my bundles leaked tobacco. As I fumbled with my prayer bags, both Merley and his sister came over and welcomed me and thoughtfully remembered and inquired about my children.

Once we'd converted our prayers to hand-held objects, we carried them to a large stick that was arrayed with various implements. The skull of a large animal, perhaps a buffalo or cow, crowned the top. It seemed to be an altar. Feathers, gems, knives and objects I wasn't sure of were attached or lying near the base. A few people added things, but we continued to hang onto our prayer bags. Merley came before us and sang some Native American prayer songs and then prayed in English for the earth, the animals, the sky, the water, just about everything I could think of, and then for each of us and all of our relations. He took a few puffs off an unusually long ceremonial pipe and addressed the four directions and the earth and sky by word and gesture. Then he had us enter the sweat through a very small opening on our hands and knees. The small conical room was constructed of willow branches and heavy tarps. I felt like a kid going into a really neat fort. As we crossed the threshold, each person repeated a prayer for all of their relations. Before the darkness of the closing of the flap, we were able to tie our bags onto supporting willow branches over our heads.

When the flap came down, I had a feeling somewhere between anticipation and apprehension. It was tight and incredibly warm, and black inside except for the surreal glow of the lava rocks in the center. You really couldn't back very far away from the rocks before touching the rim of the structure. Still, I had to use my body awareness to sense where others were because my eyes weren't doing the trick. The heat intensified rapidly and soon someone was pouring water onto the glowing rocks. I smelled sage as the steam hit my lungs like I was leaning over a humidifier in a tent on the equator.

Merley sang and prayed and occasionally spoke of our connection and responsibility to the earth and all its inhabitants. Being a group experience, others were singing, playing instruments, praying and occasionally passing the pipe around. Once in awhile, a big wooden ladle of cool water would come around for a sip. I tried to observe as much as I could, since I wasn't aware of the protocol, but mainly I steeled my will to last through at least one round. I did entertain the idea of quietly exiting until I realized I'd have to stumble over Merley to get out. I was occasionally distracted from my anxiety with a sensory display or rock-like sprinkles being thrown into the fire, which suddenly brightened and let off a pleasing aroma of cedar.

My senses were on high alert from the get-go. The occasional visuals, aromas and rhythmic singing were gratifying, but the intensity of the heat and intermittent, unexpected high-pitched voices hinted at the possibility of danger. I found it difficult to get into the meditative mood I'd anticipated, because it was taking all my energy to hold down the panic I was feeling about not being able to suck down enough air. I was sweltering. My clothes were wringing wet and I believe I may have even been panting before the end of the first round. I didn't have the focus for praying, but could feel the prayers all around, forming a current to push me onward. I finally became so exhausted I had to lie down, my stomach and face to the dirt. "The earth is my mother," I thought. "I will just rest on her for awhile." I'd never really felt the earth in such a personal way before.

After awhile the flap was opened and cold air rushed in, and for a few moments I had my chance to escape, but I couldn't get it together fast enough and then the flap was down again. There were four rounds in all, possibly lasting a few hours apiece. Time was impossible to calculate and steadily losing its relevance. At some point I began letting go of making efforts. Either I will live or die but I must stop struggling, I thought. The physical challenge was far greater than I had imagined. As my internal struggles lessened, I became more aware of something else, perhaps the body of the ritual, carrying me along.

Toward the end I was lying down without getting up anymore. I felt a strong and steady pulse coming up from the earth into my body. I recall thinking my heart should be pounding against the earth but it felt reversed. Before I'd completely abandoned effort, I'd shamelessly dug a little burrow to nest down into the cooler ground. When this brought little relief, I'd rolled to the edge of the taut tarp and tried to scratch a pit underneath so I could cheat for air. When I met with no success again, I finally surrendered completely. "This is it," I thought, and made no more attempts to save myself. I became more of an observer than an actor. It was like, "She's having a hard time breathing," instead of "Oh my god, I can't breathe!"

Then I became aware of something large moving around and sniffing from the other side of the tarp. It stopped directly across from my face. I could hear and feel its breath coming through the tarp into my mouth. I recall thinking how odd but fortunate that some dog had come to rescue me, perhaps having sensed my distress and exact location from the opposite side of the tarp. In any case, I could clearly sense and feel the animal inches from me, steadily breathing into my face. It kept me from hyperventilating as I slowed my breathing to match the pace of the large animal's breath. There was no question that it was giving me breath and teaching me how to breathe. Focusing on the steady deep breaths I heard and felt coming into my nose and mouth may have prevented me from losing consciousness.

I made it through all four rounds. When the flap was lifted for the last time, I crawled out without panic or signs of debilitation. Instead of feeling like I had overcome something, I felt like I had aligned with something. I now believe there are levels of consciousness that we can become aware of only at the point of complete surrender. When the self is too big you cannot see beyond it. Before, when I would think of ritual, I'd picture people wearing masks or specific garments in order to "play" a different role, hiding or suspending their true identities. It was a mere swapping of roles and therefore still illusory. But now I'm thinking rituals that involve role-playing have the same potential for real transformation. The taking up of costumes or masks makes visible the malleability of self. Just as change can occur in the visible world, so it can in the invisible realm of consciousness.

When the Pope is presented to the Catholic world, he looks the right way and behaves in the expected manner with all the right props. I think it gets both him and his audience in the "mood" for God. If he appeared in a stained bathrobe, smoking a cigar and waved from a rusted, sputtering jalopy, would he have the same power? I would like to say yes but I think no, because the collective mood or archetype would be compromised. Similarly, if I was just sweating in a hut, without the prayers, songs, incense and form of the ritual, would I have extended myself, or just gotten up and left when the suffering was too threatening? Knowing I was involved in ritual kept me going, and beyond that I think the collective mood of the participants added to the energy I needed. I believe more is involved in ritual than considerations of self and group. There is energy in the form itself, from centuries of use. In the case of the sweat, I was pushed beyond the boundaries of self. By self I mean everything following "my" … my body, my fears, my family, my expectations, my experience. At the point of giving these up, I became aware of something else. Perhaps anyone could become the mouthpiece of God or Goddess or higher self, if they realized the thing to dissolve is the fixed idea of "myself." Whether we need ritual or not to achieve this, I don't know. But ritual can be used as a means of expanding perception.

When I crawled out of the sweat, the sky was alive with glistening constellations. The wind in the trees and the sparks and heat from the fire were experienced directly instead of being the background of something

I was doing. Everything in the night was vivid and valid, and I was grateful to be part of it. I shivered in my wet clothes in the cold air but I felt a lightness of body that I can only describe as a lessening of gravity. I remember thinking if I leaped up I could gently float back down like an astronaut on the moon. After all, I had felt the heartbeat of the earth. I had lost my boundaries.

A cold bucket of water was brought to each of us to douse ourselves with. I thought it was just to rinse off the sweat, but a warm shower would have been kinder. I think the shock of the cold water was really to sever the tie to the ritual, to pull us back from the threshold. After I poured the cold water over my body and wrapped a towel around myself, I stood before the fire feeling very clean and alert. We soon made our way up from the canyon on a dirt trail toward Merley's house. After changing into dry clothes we gathered in a kitchen filled with plates of food and bottles of water. I was surprised to find myself neither hungry nor thirsty. I felt deeply relaxed and content.

I parked myself in a chair and observed people eating and socializing with a calm sort of interest. Normally I feel uncomfortable in group situations, but I was just fine being there, not feeling like I had to be or do anything particular. I accepted a plate of food when it was offered and soon was marveling at the exquisite depths of taste in a bite of banana. A salad and a piece of bread produced a symphony of flavor I could never properly express my gratitude towards. Water became a cool silvery balm in my system.

Merley came over and asked if there was anything I'd like to share about the experience. I laughed. I was incapable of verbalizing my experience. He seemed to understand and started to move away. "Um…" I called at his back, "where's your dog?" He turned around, looking perplexed by my question, "No dogs are allowed to come around during the sweats." "Oh," I turned back to my plate, freeing him to move onto someone who might have something insightful to say. It was words I think that broke the spell and brought me to "my" self. Could a stray dog have come along that only I knew about? Had I hallucinated? Would people think I was crazy or made it up if I related my experience? I was back to myself alright, and now I was ready to leave. When I left the house I glanced around for the dog who had saved me, but I didn't see any trace of a dog.

After sleeping like a log all night, I awoke with the same unusually sharp senses I had experienced after crawling out of the sweat. In addition, my hands and feet had an extremely warm, vibrating, highly sensitive feeling, just short of pain. It was a skinless kind of feeling, as if there were no barriers between my palms and soles and the air and ground. This sensation lasted for several days.

The day following the sweat, I felt a simmering vibe between the ground and my tingling feet as I walked on a high mountain trail. My back felt like the place where a stove door had opened, and the sensation of heat emanating from my body was not diminished by the cold icy wind against it. A close friend and I had climbed to the peak of a mountain in Laguna with his seriously depressed daughter. It had been a challenge just to get her out of the house and into my car. He prodded her up the trail like a shepherd and I tried to stay alert for dangers of stumbling and falling, but the vibrating heat was so profound that it was hard to stay focused. He meant for us to do an impromptu healing ceremony because, as we spoke on the phone that morning, he claimed to have seen her spirit leaning out of her. Being Native American, he had some ideas about bringing her back and wanted to make use of my freshly charged energy.

We lit some sage and prayed for her strength to return, each of us holding her limp hands to form a small circle. My hands felt like they were blowing heat against the cold hands of my companions. I could feel it in waves pulsing around the circle. As we walked off the mountain, my friend's daughter gradually became animated, losing the dull stare and robot-like movements. By the time we were approaching their house, she began talking coherently. I checked on her for days and she was her old self again. In fact, this was years ago and she has never regressed to depression since. Whether it was the shock of the icy wind, the concentration of prayer or the residual effects of the sweat, reignited through this impromptu ritual, that created a healing space, I cannot say.

214

I later told my friend about the dog incident at the sweat. He grinned with delight, "It wasn't a dog!"

"Of course it was a dog. I could hear it moving around and breathing, just like a very large dog."

"It was a bear!" he laughed, as if he knew something I didn't.

Well, everybody knows the bears have long since departed these lands, and I was adamant that it was a physical being, not some airy vision I'd experienced. He remained convinced, for some reason, that it had been a bear. "You'll see," he smiled, as I rolled my eyes and shook my head.

About a month later, my young daughter began having trouble with her second-grade teacher. It was getting to the point where she was having to stay after school several days a week for various infractions... not paying attention, forgetting homework, etc. My normally happy child was becoming anxious and withdrawn. I worked both ends trying to find a solution, but the problem continued to deepen. I waited for it to sort itself out. The teacher's attitude towards my daughter was becoming increasingly intolerant, but I couldn't convince her to change her tactics. My daughter began to dread going to school. She seemed permanently in trouble now. I was lying awake nights worrying.

Then I had the most vivid dream I ever had. I saw my daughter across a crowded sea of people that separated us on the school playground. To my horror, she was dangling dangerously from a high bar on the top of some playground equipment. She was going to fall and nobody noticed. There were too many and in the way. Not a chance I could get there in time to save her.

Suddenly I felt something shift and a sensation of power filled me. I could see, smell and hear everything with a piercing sharpness. I bent low and set my palms on the ground and felt heat coming up through the grass as my hands and feet thickened. My nails lengthened and became hard and sharp, easily penetrating to the dirt beneath the grass. I looked up and saw the crowd as shapes of obstacles and scanned for weak spots in the barrier. Sensing the proper direction, I took off like lightning, zigzagging towards my target on all fours. In a flash, my perspective split as I watched from above and simultaneously bounded towards my daughter in the shape of a running bear. The dream abruptly ended as I caught my daughter in time, back in my human shape.

I woke up exhilarated, knowing that I had the power to save my daughter. It inspired me to go to the school and speak directly to the principal about the conflict. My previous hesitations about appearing as an interfering or ignorant parent of an unruly child had vanished. My kid needed a mother bear, for crying out loud. As I stepped into the principal's office, I felt some anxiety creeping back, but I quickly focused on the sensations of the dream bear. Instead of trivializing the situation as I expected, the principal immediately agreed the teacher was out of line. The situation that had caused so much grief was neutralized that very day.

I realize these unusual incidents could be explained away by skeptics as hallucinations and coincidence, but they each preceded actual positive results in my life. Truth can be felt through experience, or assumed by detached intellectual methods. I choose sensory involvement in my measure of reality. Something transformative happened to me, provoked by the ritual of the Native American sweat. Somewhere between my fears of annihilation and my awakening to a deeply nurturing energy, I was transported to a larger field of possibilities.

Wedding the Underworld

Thomas A. Habib

The wedding party gathered on a fine June afternoon at the base of the Park City Deer Valley Mountain Ski Resort. A white runner decorated with purple flower petals lay upon the grass, dividing the two families soon to be united. Large umbrellas provided some respite from a summer sun destined to lose its intensity in the months ahead. The thickly treed mountain, with huge swaths of ski trails cut through it, dwarfed the ensemble assembled and loomed over this young couple's untested love.

I noticed Janel dabbing at the tears in her eyes. Some she missed began to fall upon her bouquet. A glistening trickle of tears grew into an avalanche as she turned her head away, perhaps ashamed, and sobbed into the mountain. Many in attendance had gathered just two short weeks earlier to bury her groom's brother. While this usually happy occasion had been months in the planning, the sobering shadow of death was close to the surface for many of us, now released by Janel.

The groom's parents softly cried . . . an exhausted and spent cry, long past any possible Faustian bargaining.

A wave of sadness infiltrated the gathering. I began to cry with others. We were joined by death and love that knows no cultural boundaries. I felt the beloved in the other . . . for Janel, for my brother-in-law and sister-

217

in-law, and for all of the guests.

Vows were exchanged and the wedding proceeded through the recessional, "Ode to Joy." The newly wedded couple greeted the guests for the first time as husband and wife. Janel apologized for her tears. I wanted to hug her. I felt love. My gratitude was to grow later as I realized that she helped us remember ancient wisdoms: that time is finite, change must be expected, and death inevitable.

On the lodge veranda before to the formal reception in the shadow of the mountain, many cried and hugged. Word circulated that the restroom was full of tearful women. My nephew died alone late at night, in his car in his parents' driveway, at 31 years of age. I couldn't stop sobbing, and tried to hide in the crevice of my wife's back. Death was supposed to be a slow process that culminated in one's elderly years.

This was not going to be easy. My usual emotional comfort zone was to live like Prometheus and rip a piece of the fire from the Gods. The magic of Merlin or the Trickster's elusiveness, from which I often drew, could not immunize me this time. I knew the Sage would return later-- time was liminal. But all of us were being rescaled, with the possibility of later finding something closer to our essential purpose (Houston, 2004). Wounding like this can be a doorway to a larger world.

When the reception began we were able to laugh during the best man's toast and warm to the bridal waltz. The ebb and flow of disparate feelings during these times would lead to a new reorganization. When the courageous decision was made to proceed with this wedding, the shadow of death was an invited guest. Mortality defines our humanity. It creates "leaky margins" (Houston, 1996) in a world where too often we become forgetful., where forgetfulness costs us our mindfulness. To gain wisdom, one must listen to the wild dogs in our cellar, as Nietzsche told us. A plutonic grounding is what keeps us from forgetting that this time could abruptly end.

The dancing began as the last hint of light faded behind the mountain, now in shadow. A canopy of stars sparked those of us who stepped off of the dance floor into the cool alpine air to raise our gaze in awe. "These times do not last forever" I said to an elder named Dallas from Atlanta as we watched these tribes, mostly from Vermont and Utah, pound the dance floor with passion and resolve. In shared collective radiance for life , we were alive and celebrating an expanding family. A waiter, who had undoubtedly seen many weddings, remarked how much fun the people were having.

I am en route to still another family wedding as I write the story of a wedding unlike any I've ever attended. Rarely doo we witness pain and joy so closely aligned. Many of the same family that joined the reality of death together that June afternoon will be in attendance. I will look for signs of how their stories have been rewritten. I wish for them the many jewels that one can mine from such a journey with Hermes through the underworld. During these journeys, one does not stop short by notice of pain, but rather grow by savoring the unfolding story. I can only hope that we remain mindful of the time we have, the love we share, the ever-present choice to feel grateful. Mindful that significance is more important than success, we can unburden from trying to make a favorable impression, and know the divine within. To take this path, we will honor the wounds of experience and remain faithful to the communion we share.

References:
Houston, Jean. Jump Time. Shaping Your Future in a World of Radical Change. Sentient Publications 2004.

Houston, Jean. A Mythic Life: Learning to Live Our Greater Story. Harper One 1996.

A Desert Fast

John Davis

I AM EXPOSED ON HIGH GROUND AT THE NORTH END OF A LONG, NARROW desert valley. A light wind comes off the mountains to the north, and the full length of the valley sweeps away below me. It's October – hot days, cold nights. I have been alone, fasting from food and drinking only water, for the past four days. With the end of the fourth day approaching, I have prepared for an all-night vigil in a small circle of stones and sticks. This ceremony, a wilderness rite of passage or vision fast, provides the outline and structure for my solo fast and my vigil: four days of preparation and severance from my familiar life, four days of solitude without food and with only a minimum of shelter. Time for reincorporation and integration will come later. The structure of the ceremony and the support of my guides are profound, but with the arrival of the last night of my solo, I am increasingly alone.

As the setting sun pauses for a moment on the western mountains, I put my sleeping bag, ground pad, and water bottle into the circle. Slowly, I take off my clothes and place them into the circle. I say a prayer for strength through the night, hoping for a vision of my place in the world and guidance for my work as a wilderness guide. As the sun dips below the horizon, I bow to say good-bye and step into the circle. My aim is to stay here all night, awake. Once in the circle, I quickly put my clothes back on; it is cold now.

I have fasted in a similar way several times before this and received deep, strong teachings and insights. This time is different, however. I have deliberately set higher goals for myself. Not knowing exactly what I need,

I sense that the more I can let go, the more I will get out of it. My mantra the last four days has been "Dig Deeper."

Another difference is symbolized by going naked into the circle. I am seeking as much openness as possible. In the past, I went into my vigils with my meditation beads, journal, Tibetan cymbals, songs, chants, and other tools for awakening. This time I leave all that behind, taking only what I feel I need for safety during the night. Going naked represents my intention to simply be here, just me in the circle. In parallel, my intention for the solo has been simplifying, almost like the sun and wind blowing away my wishes and hopes until nothing but the bones of my intention remain. The question I couldn't quite voice goes something like this: "Do I have what I need to live my life?"

As the night comes on, stars appear in the east and the blue in the west deepens. Shooting stars come down, some on the edge of my awareness, some full-bore in front of me, leaving fantastic blue trails. Like sweets, they delight me. I sit in my circle for a while, and when my legs get tired, I move around the circle in a slow, shuffling dance. From time to time, I stretch and bow, usually to nothing in particular.

I have been trying not to have too many expectations about a "vision," but it is hard. How often have I told others not to expect any particular kind of vision? "A vision can come in many different forms; be open to whatever happens, including nothing." But I find it hard to let go of my expectations. Instead, I let them surface, all the hopes and fears. Maybe animals will speak to me or the sky will open to reveal a chorus of angels, maybe not. What if nothing at all happens? Maybe, this is my biggest fear – emptiness, insignificance, pointlessness.

At first, I have lots of energy, but as the night comes on I find myself more tired. The past few days, my energy went from high and even agitated in the beginning to exhaustion and on to a quiet, clean, and impeccable clarity through my mind and body. My hunger peaked in the second day, and now I barely notice it. During the last day of the solo, I felt as if my body-mind were a clear bottle which has been scrubbed clean from inside.

I move and stretch often during the first part of the night. I try meditating, but my mind is uncooperative. It seems to be jerking around a lot, bouncing, even frantic. Feeling that I need to do something with the incessant thinking, I decide I will give my mind something useful to do—or at least something it's good at. I'll let it do calculations. The waxing quarter moon has been up for some time. I measure various angles and, according to some formula I can't remember now, I figure that when the moon sets, dawn will be just a couple hours away. Judging from how high the moon is in the night sky, dawn won't be long now. I settle down for the remaining few hours of night with a growing sense of completion. The night is still getting colder and I wrap myself in my sleeping bag. "This hasn't been too difficult," my mind comments with relief.

I spend more time sitting, shuffling, or jumping up and down. It is a struggle to stay awake, but I am working at it. I count more shooting stars, I hum softly to myself, and I make myself conscious of my breathing. At one point, the world stops. There is a timeless moment of total stillness and silence, deep, black, and peaceful. I am conscious of the stillness, unlike sleep, and I am aware of the lack of mental activity other than this bare recognition and knowing. The moment feels total, complete, and infinite.

Soon enough, the stillness is replaced by more mental activity, some of it downright rowdy. For example, I find myself going around to my favorite restaurants ordering meals. It doesn't matter that the food never comes, just ordering is enough. ("I'll have samosas for an appetizer, the chicken curry, onion naan bread, and rice pudding for desert. ... Swiss cheeseburger with slaw and extra tomato, fries, and a beer ... Rice and veggies, water to drink, no ice.").

My calculations have been off, however. When I figure dawn is just over the horizon, the night is still deepening. It is now much longer than I had planned. It is very difficult to stay awake and focused. My mind is running around like crazy. My body aches. I am almost too tired to move, but I know if I stop for more than a minute I will drop off to sleep. I need my sleeping bag for warmth, but it threatens to seduce me into sleep. I feel so tempted to step outside my circle back to the soft sand of the last three nights and sleep.

It is no longer a vigil for a vision but just a struggle to stay in my circle and stay awake. The night stretches on like this. It should be dawn by now! I seriously consider the possibility that some crazy cosmic catastrophe has brought the world into continuous night and the dawn will never come. Yes, seriously. I give up all hope except my intention of staying awake in my circle. Finally, finally, however, the dark in the east softens almost imperceptibly. I breathe a sigh of relief, and I find I am crying. I know the night still has a long way to go, but at least it is moving.

The sun breaks the horizon. I whoop with joy, I say a prayer to the sun, and I take a moment before stepping outside my circle. I feel great relief but oddly also a hint of disappointment and even defeat. Now, though, it is time to pack my stuff up, disappear my circle, and meet my buddy. Activity fills me, and the feeling of disappointment recedes. It is good to see my buddy. The guides who stayed at basecamp greet me with smiles, simple prayers, sage incense, and hugs. It truly feels good to be in their arms and to see the others. I am quiet and open, and the warm sun is delicious. The food tastes exquisite. ("I'll have fresh fruit and a cup of herb tea.") I also offer prayers for those who are hungry without choice.

The next two days, I spend much of my time listening to others' stories as my teachers work with them. I am not talking much about my experiences. Since I will be around for another week, they focus on those who need to return to their daily lives. However, in quiet moments, my sense of failure is growing. I am feeling that I wasted a once-in-a-lifetime opportunity. Instead of going into a profound state or opening myself to some great insight, I just hung out thinking about food and trying to get comfortable. The skies never opened to reveal Truth, no animals whispered my name, and I struggled. Something grates on me about not having been graceful and centered throughout the night. I let go of anything subtle or esoteric, and I just scratched around in the dirt, waiting for the night to end. I groveled in my little circle. I groveled! I catch the odor of old shame, the shame of being insignificant and needy, the shame that my time in the ceremony had been pointless.

***

It is now the third day following my fast, I am sleeping in the sage flats outside of the desert town where my teachers live. My campsite is very plain, and to me, very beautiful. It's just a patch of bare ground surrounded by low bushes. Songbirds flit through, and I have a stunning view of the mountains across the valley. Waking in the cool air before dawn, a very strong sense fills me – crystal clear and sharp as a rising sun. Now I get it! The simple, undeniable fact is that I did everything I set out to do on my ceremony. I went into my circle on the fourth night of a solo fast in the desert, I stayed in that circle through the night, I stayed awake, and I stepped back out of that circle. No long, involved story and no dramatic emotional catharsis, just a simple, certain truth.

However simple it is, though, its impact on me is profound. Still in my sleeping bag, I feel I buoyed up, held in some greater arms. How can I can continue to deny my own capacity? I was truly exposed in that circle. It was hard, and I really struggled! And I did what I set out to do. The fullness and completeness I feel is not a sense of personal accomplishment against something nor a sense of winning, but rather a sense that these events have taken place through me. I feel humble and grateful, and my heart is more relaxed than I have known.

All my images and idealizations evaporated in the unbounded, eternal darkness of that desert night. Avoiding neediness and struggle had kept me from a deeper sense of my own capacity. Needing to look good, even if I was the only one around, had been at my ideal. Yet, on my vigil, that had all cracked open. What emerged was my actual experience. I had groveled and yet, I had completed my intention for that ceremony. I had done what I set out to do. Gracefulness be damned. Indeed, my life is big enough to include groveling, too.

The lesson of that vision fast in the desert is that I hold within me-- and I can open myself to-- all that I need. This is enough. Lying there in the sage flats, taking in the cool air, and watching the dawn, I remember a passage from Castaneda's **Tales of Power** in which Don Juan tells Carlos:

You say you need help. Help for what? You have everything needed for the extravagant journey that is your life. I have tried to teach you that the real experience is to be a man and that what counts is being alive; life is the little detour that we are taking now. Life in itself is sufficient, self-explanatory, and complete.

I now have an answer to the question I brought to my fast. "Do I have what I need to live my life?" Yes, I do. I confirmed that in the ceremony of the solo. I am held, even when I struggle, and I am capable even when I fall apart. This sense of capacity is not dependent on my meeting any standards or being any particular way. It's in the nature of being alive and awake in the singular and unique circle of my life. Meanwhile, the sun's warmth releases smells of the sage, and sparrows flit noisily from bush to bush. Time now for breakfast. "Granola with almonds and raisins and a cup of black tea, please."

ASHES, ASHES, WE ALL FALL DOWN

PETER RIORDAN

OUR INTIMATE GROUP OF TEN SETTLED IN AROUND THE FIRE-PIT. THE visiting Huichol *marakame* (shaman) began the fire ceremony. The Huichol (pronounced wee-chol) refer to themselves as Wixarika, not Huichol, which is a misnomer dragged through centuries of speculation about their origin. Are they descended from the Guachichils, the Chichimecs, the Toltecs? Are they forebears of the Aztecs? Their language is said to be closely related to the Hopi tongue of the American southwest, with whom they share similarities in their relationships with god and evidence of shared ancient trade routes. This aloof culture has amazingly survived fairly intact, despite many conquests, domestic and foreign, including the Spanish conquest and ensuing missionary system.

"Was there danger in making eye contact with the marakame during the ceremony?" I wondered, as I strove to engage the fire flashing in his dark eyes. Chanting and singing without hesitation, from the heart, as he engaged the spirit world through his magic portal, *nierica*. I didn't understand the language, but the vibe was overwhelming, the emotion, raw and spontaneous. I looked around our circle and no one seemed to be making eye contact.

Apathetic and mute
I struggle to hear the music
Distant and muffled

The indigenous rhythms
Ethereal, dreamlike . . .
Coming closer . . . Clearer
Appearing now, feathers aflutter
Fetish dancing in his hand
Directing a rhythmic cadence
The portal opens, nierica achieved
The sing-song voice now resonant
Hypnotizing
Praising, praying, warning
Pleading, crying, laughing
Simultaneously
Laser-like interpretations
Bridging primal and modern
Conscious and unconscious
Awakening . . .
I hear the shaman sing!

The song lasted for about an hour, although we were told that the marakame will go on for many hours without interruption. He then addressed each of us individually and through an interpreter gave us personal advice. I was told to spend less time on the computer. We'd never met; I am a graphic designer who spends many hours daily on the computer. He also told me that Mother Nature was sick and needed our help.

At the end of the ceremony the marakame blessed the place of the fire pit, leaving an ally (translated if in this dimension it would look something like a butterfly) for the surround. He said that in a few days all would be changed.

Hot Santa Ana winds were building, showing promise of kicking up, as we thanked our host said good night. My fiancée and I drove the short mile home. I turned on the sprinklers to soak the property down due to the hot, dry winds, and we went to bed. The winds grew stronger overnight. Awakened a few times to the fierce howling. Our house was perched on a western rim overlook of the valley 200' below.

The genesis of the Witch Creek Fire was just a mile up the road from the previous evening's ceremony. Generated by record Santa Ana winds, a heat wave, an on-going drought, tinder dry chaparral, the sparks from the wind-blown power-line quickly became an out of control wildfire. The Witch Creek Fire consumed 197,990 acres, 1,040 homes, including our hosts' and our own.

With a great swath of her brush
The landscape is all different
Mother Nature demands change.

Charred skeletal forest casting fantastic shapes
Against the ash strewn, sandy soil
Huge boulders emerge, blackened
Surreal backdrop of what was home.

My lookout much less shaded than before
Gazing into the valley 200' below
There! The unmistakable silhouette of a puma
Dashing, momentarily exposed
Along the tree line of the seasonal stream
Long tail, ruddering her long sinuous, sensuous strides
Gone in an instant!

Coyotes still howl here at night
How did they survive?
I watch as a red-tailed hawk leaps into flight
Screeching off its', boulder top perch . . .
Soaring up and away

Maybe with all the chaparral burned away
That old mine entrance will be exposed
Or a bobcat or mountain lion den

Heavy redwood plank
Notched to fit the gnarly trunks
of the old twin oaks.
You missed my bench here . . . Ha-ha!
All consuming monster,

The Great Witch Creek Fire is out!

The aloe is blooming.

The experience coalesced transformation forces to the extreme, -- raging fire, raging weather, raging earth and sky with great personal loss, pain and suffering. I have been majestically and mercifully guided to witness Nature's re-birth. I've hiked through the fire ravaged canyons of the Cleveland National Forest most days since the fires of October 2007. The growth literally from out of the ashes has been nothing short of miraculous. It is proving to be a catalyst for deep personal and positive change. Instead of losses, I see renewal, providing hope, growth, and a personal intimacy with Creation in ways I've never experienced.

Perhaps it is self-centered to think that there is symbiosis between the shamans' presence, his fire ceremony, and the ensuing wildfire. How could something we were so intimately involved with be so interrelated? Yet, I wonder, what of greater importance was taking place within those moments with the singing shaman, that could/would have such an effect?

Not loss, but sacrifice!

My 7.2 pound Zen Master

MELIS ALKIN

I HAD ALWAYS LOOKED UP TO THOSE WHO WERE DISCIPLINED ENOUGH to have a *practice*. Natalie Goldberg had a writing practice, Ken Wilber woke up at dawn to meditate. Leonard Cohen, who constantly moved back and forth between a life of cigarettes and music and poetry to the monastery, had sufficient discipline to become a monk. Then there are the professionals in my field who practice mindfulness and meditation, who with calmness and pride talk about their use of ritualized practices. I knew that within all of these stories that there had to be some healing in following a mindful practice. I secretly wished that I had found myself a Zen master who would force me to follow *the path*. But whether from fear or procrastination, I never looked for one.

That unfinished search ended when I had a baby. Nursing, diaper change, and sleep routines *became* my practice. You have to feed a newborn every three hours or so and comfort her to sleep multiple times a day and night. Absolutely no other ritual can be this forceful, healing, and bonding-- with the survival of another being at its core. It is physical, emotional, spiritual, relational, and continuous.

My master did not allow for any distractions, especially when she was nursing. I held my daughter in my arms to nurse or comfort her to sleep for countless hours. The image of this picture is supposed to be that of peace and love, but the reality of such a selfless ritual is a lot more complicated than that.

The *self* often gets in the way. It sometimes wants to take a break or just do something else for a change. Even if you willingly put everything else on hold, the list of wants moves from items of pleasure to basic necessity: from "I want to watch a movie, read a book, wash the dishes, do laundry, take a shower" to "I *really* need to sleep, pee, eat or drink some water".

For the most part, remembering my short-term attempts at meditating, I was able to follow the mantra "acknowledge the thought (or the need) and just it let go" in order to stay in a physically uncomfortable position for what seemed like eternity. Other times I temporarily lost my equanimity, and even thought I was even losing my mind. For me, those moments of hardship came as a blow to my newly established confidence. And my master would change the rules of the rituals just when I thought to have figured them out.

During those moments of insanity, crying because my patience was depleted, I wondered why I could not stay a little longer and why it was so difficult to impose a discipline on a mind that equally sought love, connection, grounding, and freedom.

One of the first lessons involved the impermanent quality of my daily routines. I bought one of the parenting books about sleep solutions for babies. I read the whole book, which included multiple tricks to put your baby to sleep and even teach them how to fall asleep by themselves. I tried all the possible techniques and gave them up one after the other, since my master was adamant to keep to her preferred methods of sleeping. By the time I was completing that book, and had just had come to accept that I was a failure at this task, the author wrote that the most peaceful method for babies to sleep was to be held and nursed, and that mothers should cherish those moments as long as they could.

My 7.2 pound master had started to teach me that, for the most part, I too could experience the healing of soul through discipline-- relational rituals practiced whether lying down, nursing, sitting on a bench at a park, or repetitive playing for countless hours.

I realized that I was pushing too hard to go with what came naturally. The culprit was partly the parenting books, but mostly it was my pre-established habits, with my focus on getting things done, on time.

I learned to cherish those relational (sometimes peaceful) moments as a blessing and a teaching, and to put life and priorities into perspective. Those first years with my Master became the foundation of a life-practice of grounding and surrendering to *being*.

INTO THE LION'S DEN: A TRANSDANCE RITE OF PASSAGE

ALISHA LENNING SOLAN

The roaring of lions, the howling of wolves, the raging of the stormy sea, and the destructive sword, are portions of eternity, too great for the eye
--William Blake

Like all vibrant elements of nature, human beings grow in the light and transform in the dark. -- Wilbert Alix

TranceDance is a neo-shamanic ritual developed by Wilbert Alix and the Natale Institute. Alix describes neo-shamanism as a modern re-working of cross-cultural impulses. For Alix (2007), an important aspect of neo-shamanism is that it creates new rituals, rather than merely "hijacking" rituals from indigenous cultures. TranceDance incorporates the following elements of ritual that show up in many different traditional cultures: dance, darkness, drumming, and trance as a potential spiritual and healing state. TranceDance also adds modern elements, such as recorded music, surround-sound stereos, and the notions of individuality, shadow work, and personal responsibility. I have practiced TranceDance for many years, and one of my most dramatically transformative experiences relates to writing my doctoral dissertation.

TranceDance follows a classic ritual structure of Separation, Transition, and Return (Achterberg, 1994, p. 22). In the Separation phase, TranceDancers *set an intention* and *put on a blindfold* to enter the privacy of darkness and to shut out ordinary reality. During my doctoral TranceDance, I set my intention to resolve the conflicted feelings I had about completing my degree. I tied the bandana around my eyes, to shut out the world of conflicting obligations: the university, an academically "war-torn" department, my parents, my partner, the ongoing financial pressures of graduate school.

I began the double-inhale breath of TranceDance, moving my body to the rhythm of the music in order to enter the Transition phase of "shamanic trance" where *music, movement, and breath* stimulate TranceDancers to open themselves to a 60-75 minute "trance state" or "inner journey" that may go beyond normal perceptions of space, time, and identity. Alix (2007) describes "shamanic trance" as using repetitive rhythm to get the body to enter a "state of entrainment" where the mind does not need to be engaged in regulating the body. Thus, the consciousness can "journey" away from the body and is free to fly over "inner landscapes" (from author's notes). And so, my consciousness flew:

First, I am a hunter, stalking a deer in the forest. I hide in the bush, creeping ever closer. I release my arrow and bring down a buck. I carry the heavy animal over my shoulder for miles, weeping. Finally I find a spot that feels right to set my burden down. I offer the deer up to the heavens. I offer myself up. Then, I draw a knife and carve into the buck's flesh; my hands grow sticky, warm and bloodied. The deer's antlers become a headdress, and blood mingles with tears on my face.

In my new garb, I continue my journey with a greater sense of desperation. I run for miles and miles. I run through the desert. I run through the jungle. I run for days and nights, nights and days. A thunderstorm arises, but I continue to run through sheets of water and mud.

At last, I arrive at shelter-- a cave. I enter the cave, breathing hard. The cave is dark, and I can see nothing but blackness. Then, gradually, I make out the shape of golden figures all around me. I have entered the cave of lion's den. I am surrounded by lions on all sides. Before me, the lead-male--a large, well-maned animal-- sits on a dais. I bow my head to the ground in supplication. When I look up again, the lion leaps. He leaps at me, open-mouthed. He leaps into me. He swallows me whole. This image of the lion's leap repeats itself over and over again in instant replay, like a game-winning touchdown on television.

Eventually, I sense the time for me to leave the cave. I exit through the back way, down a different tunnel than I'd come in. The tunnel grows narrower and narrower as I move forward until I have to crawl on my hands and knees to pass through. Ahead, the tunnel forks into two distinct paths. I am aware, even in this trance state, that the two paths before me represent my two choices: to complete my degree or to leave it behind and quit. I take a breath and chose the path of completion. I follow my chosen path as it grows wider and wider. Finally, it leads me out of the cave and into the wash of rain that now feels exhilarating. I dance a celebratory dance. Then, from outside I hear the sound that heralds the end of the TranceDance ritual. I lie down on the ground, and allow myself to be called back to ordinary reality.

In the Return phase of TranceDance, an "ohm" sound calls Trance-Dancers to lie on the floor for 5-15 minutes, allowing the body to rest and the spirit to return. Then, the TranceDancers remove their bandanas and gather into a circle where facilitators and other dancers support each other to ground back to ordinary reality. In the circle, TranceDancers are invited to share their journey experiences, if they so desire, before returning to their ordinary lives. I joined the circle of other TranceDancers, and we shared our experiences. When I went home, I slept deeply. That night, I felt healed.

Now, I wish I could say that I woke up the next morning with the perfect dissertation topic clearly outlined in my head. I wish I could say that the battle in my department ended with no casualties. I wish I could say that I was awarded a huge fellowship grant that allowed me to quit all my part-time work and focus on my writing. But indeed, these and other challenges still remained.

Healing does not necessarily relieve us of our problems. In fact, as Jeanne Achterberg notes, healing can even create problems and crises to induce deeper healing. She describes a healing ritual as:

any ritual whose purpose is to make whole--the root word of healing is *hale*, or "to make whole." . . . the purpose of healing is not just to return a body or mind back to what society considers normal. Rather, the goal is to become better, more enlightened, or stronger than before the problem existed (Achterberg, 1994, p. 9).

Thus, the healing purpose of my TranceDance was not necessarily for me to write my dissertation and to graduate. Rather, its purpose was to restore my sense of wholeness and to make me a "whole" person with or without a PhD. It served to ease my spirit, and to raise my self-esteem regarding my relationship to my life. Yes, I continued to have setbacks, frustrations, and writer's blocks, but something did profoundly change on the night of that Trance Dance--me!

I found a new and stronger commitment to myself that night. I never again spoke of quitting. I stopped questioning *whether* I would write, and began to more seriously question *what* and *how* I would write. A short time later, I found a teaching assistant position at the Writing Center. This position provided financial stability, as well as inspiring interactions with other graduate students from many disciplines. By the end of that semester, I had completed my research proposal, and my committee approved my plans. The following May, I held my doctoral diploma in my hand.

The process of earning a degree is a ritual unto itself. The dissertation is the final challenge in an arduous cultural rite of passage from student to expert. When I coach graduate students through the dissertation process, I encourage my clients to use other more personal rituals to help them navigate this cultural rite of passage. The forms of their rituals may vary, but form is not as important as what fills it.

In this way, I see ritual as a potential space--a vessel or container for transformative possibility. Ritual is a time or space set aside through symbolic acts and attitudes that allow us to become emptied and filled anew. A full cup does not invite renewal; it is already defined, already full. But that which has been emptied can allow an infinite number of potentials to pour in and transform that emptiness. In the emptiness created by ritual, we can experience both subtle and profound healing changes beyond the realm of intellect and reason. By incorporating such rituals into the challenges of something like dissertation writing, one may earn a doctorate not only of the mind, but also of the heart or spirit. To earn such a "higher" degree, one must be willing to enter the darkness of the lion's den.

References

Achterberg, Jeanne (1994). *Rituals of healing: Using imagery for health and healing.* New York: Bantam Books.

Alix, Wilbert (April 27- May 26, 2007). TranceDance facilitator training [lecture from author's notes]. Kehena Beach, Hawaii.

The Spirit of the Carcajou

Shodai Sennin James A. Overton-Guerra

The trail up the mountain suddenly led into a thick mist that stretched before him like an ominous white curtain. Absorbed in his progress he neither paused nor contended its place but rather proceeded into it, determined to stay the course. It wasn't for quite a number of steps that he noticed the complete change of temperature and scenery to what now seemed like a different world: the warm mountain climate had been replaced by a near arctic landscape covered in snow and enshrouded in a dense and oppressive fog. His pace slowly ground to a halt as he became aware of an eerie sensation that had unexpectedly materialized within him: *fear.*

At first the feeling was a knowing impression at the periphery of his awareness and he simply ignored it, attributing it to the sudden marked change in temperature and dramatic increase in humidity that impacted his mostly naked sweaty body. Gradually the sensation intensified to the point that he had to attend to it, for fear demanded his attention.

He was quite surprised by his own thoughts, and he was not sure what they betrayed: a lack of confidence? Regret? Guilt? Loneliness? What was happening to him?? He was by himself, with himself, why would he be afraid?!? But he was; in fact he was overcome with terror. He wanted to cry out, but knew it to be both in vain and demeaning if the already pathetic feelings he was experiencing within were manifested to the cosmos. He felt small and insignificant, as if everything he ever did or could ever do would amount to little more than the silent emptiness that presently engulfed him. It was as if everything were nothing; it was as if he himself were nothing; it was as if the immensity of the universe, of nature, of this very trail and mountain he so arrogantly wished to challenge and fathom came crashing down on him all at once and crushed him in spirit if not in body. Running with Wolves! Swimming with Killer Whales! Following the Eagle, *his* Eagle in the sky! What was wrong with him? Who did he think he was? Something special? How could he have fooled himself so? How was this possible? Why had he not drowned in the depths of the bay swimming with the Orcas only to wish to cease to 'be,' here so close to the summit? What was wrong with him? Where was his Power, his warrior's Pride? Why did he suddenly break, wimp out, crumble?!?

It was in the midst of this cerebral fog that his mind barely caught a glimpse of an ephemeral shadow, a furtive blur that made him spin around in a wild-eyed panic. What was that?!? "Am I going crazy too?" he cried aloud. But as he repeatedly whirled around trying to materialize into a concrete visual image the flash he was not sure was real or a hallucination, he noticed that he was disoriented, that he no longer knew which was the path of return or where his path had been leading. He was stuck, dizzied and lost. It was at that precise instant that the first attack came.

A ripping, searing pain that shot through his body like a dagger of ice cutting him from groin to scalp stopped his very breathing. His back arched as much from the unexpected abruptness of the event as from the agony itself. Mouth agape and eyes as large as plates he instinctively spun in the direction of the attack while his brain scrambled to interpret into reality the flood of cryptic messages that his senses presented. Terror gripped him as he impulsively reached down to grasp the source of pain at his left rear flank, only to feel a hot sticky wet substance flowing liberally down his backside and now over his hand. He caught another ephemeral glimpse of a shadow as it retreated into he was not sure which direction even as his mind ran through possible supernatural explanations for what was happening. Frantically glancing around all he saw were trees and more trees fading into the white distance. Nothing made sense as terror clutched his very being, paralyzing his thought.

The second attack caught him on his right side and he distinctly felt teeth sinking into his flesh; instantly he roared in pain. Once again he swerved to get a visual on his attacker, and yet again it disappeared into the forest without a trace, like a phantom, like an invisible evil presence that left nothing but wounds, pain and terror in its wake. The attacks kept coming, now with more speed and greater frequency. His legs failed him and he collapsed onto the ground, writhing with agony, shocked that such a degree of pain was possible for he had never . . . no! Not true! A flash of memory coming from a wave of abrupt familiarity, rolled back the years to that place, to that time, and to that . . . to that helpless state as a child . . . but a child he was no more! A flicker of anger that soon became a torrent of wrath overtook him, overwhelming and overriding his agony. Nostrils flared, teeth gritted, lips curled and snarling like a raging beast, his face became a mask of wild fury as he regained his feet. No longer content to withstand and avoid, he was now determined to hunt and destroy the angry demon. As if shocked by the transition of its prey, the shadow materialized to reveal an equally snarling and fearless adversary: the bloodthirsty Carcajou!

Both opponents now circled each other in a battle to the death as the Carcajou no longer had the advantage of possession of the man's spirit and heart, but now had to fight him "mano a mano," from outside his mind and body. The man kicked and the Carcajou nimbly retreated, the beast lunged and snapped and the man leapt and dodged. Man and beast attacked and defended, neither making the least progress until suddenly the man, synchronizing his movements with those of the great *mustelid*, managed to connect a ferocious kick against the very muzzle of the beastly ghost, hurling it backwards in a head over tail tumble across the snow, shrieking like a whipped dog. This incensed the Carcajou who, wild with fury and hatred, attacked in reckless abandon, and tossing all caution to the four winds took a prodigious leap towards the man's throat. The man offered his left forearm as a shield and target for the Carcajou's furious wrath and gaping jaws. The Carcajou clenched onto the man's left forearm and both of them heard the cracking of the bones even before the man felt the shock waves of pain that quickly paralyzed his entire left side. But the warrior would not be stopped. With the lightning speed that had so often characterized him in battle, he dropped to the ground, slamming the Carcajou on its back. Stabbing his knee in its chest, he pinned it against the snow. In a continuous blood curling frenzy of human and animal snarls, of animal claws tearing and ripping human flesh, and of human flesh splattering blood in all directions, the man mercilessly beat the beast with his right fist until the Carcajou lay a limp mass of broken bones, battered meat, and flattened tissue and fur. It is doubtful that the man even registered the bones in his own hands cracking from the tremendous and relentless impact he imparted upon the skeleton of the spirit-animal.

He did not stop striking until his arm no longer responded to his will to continue, long after the carcass had relinquished its grip and its life. Chest heaving with exertion, both hands clenched in white-knuckled fists as his eyes rolled in their sockets towards the top of his head. Falling back and sitting on his heels, his head and face upturned to the sky, he emitted a primal scream of rage, desperation, and detachment to all things in a manner that seemed to howl: "This is it? This is it? This is all you have? This is what you sent to destroy me? I don't care!!! I STILL AM!!!" The roar boomed into the mist, reverberating through the trunks and branches of the forest's trees, echoing into the far-off mountains. In the distance the thunder of a great storm replied to his calling.

For moments or hours – no one knows - he sat there exhausted, emptied and full. Finally regaining himself, he felt his power surge once again, and the will to keep moving pulled him to his feet. Disoriented still, his mind delayed in recognizing, as snow the flakes, the white stuff he noticed falling from the sky. The seasoned warrior that he was, he took stock of his numerous wounds and lacerations as he remembered one of his favorite expressions: *a warrior without scars has never been to battle.* After a functional assessment of his condition, he resolved that he had no choice but to press on forward, always forward. But where, in which direction? Looking around for a sign, he noticed the figure of the Eagle, *his* Eagle, calmly resting atop a branch: he knew that to be the Way.

When he limped to where the Eagle awaited him he looked back at what he had left behind. He was stunned to see that the carcass of the Carcajou was no longer that of the mangled and broken furry beast he had left behind, but rather that of a man – himself! Even more astounding was the realization that the tracks in the snow leading from the killing ground to where he now stood were not his, nor even those of a man, but rather those of the Carcajou itself.

4

HEALING RITUALS IN PRACTICE

Surgery as Ritual

Judith J. Petry

As the High Priest performs his ablutions in the temple anteroom, the victim is prepared by assistants. Having fasted and cleansed herself, she is gently placed on an altar in the center of the temple where sacred herbs are administered to calm her and place her in a trance state. A special priest positions himself at her seventh chakra where he maintains the state of deep trance with inhaled vapours. Her clothing has been removed and replaced with specially designed and sanctified robes that outline the sacrificial site. This site is ceremonially cleansed and painted with holy oils. A bright light is focused on the site and the instruments of sacrifice are prepared in a traditional pattern by a priestess to one side of the victim.

Music that resonates with the spirit of the high priest fills the temple. When he has finished with his preparations, he enters the temple backwards with his hands outstretched before him, deterring any evil energy from entering unseen. A helper places his ceremonial robes on him, secures them and covers his hands with gloves. He places himself at the side of the victim and asks the assistant priest if the trance is deep enough to begin the ritual. The answer is yes and the high priest extends his right hand palm up and is handed the instrument of sacrifice by the assistant.

He carefully cuts open the victim's body, layer upon layer, respecting meridians and energy fields, entering her sacred center. His hands probe the physical home of her soul and find the object of sacrifice. It is separated from her life force and removed to a sacred bowl and taken from the temple. There is a feeling of jubilation in the room as the High Priest repairs the sacrificial site and calls in the energies of healing, stabilizing her life force and renewing her soul.

As the last layers of her body are reapproximated in the manner in which the gods created her, the final binding threads are placed and the site is blessed with herbs and oils, and covered with holy cloths. She is awakened from her trance and taken to an anteroom where she will recover her consciousness and begin her new life, sanctified by her sacrifice, renewed and reborn to new possibilities.

Modern surgery, a Mayan sacrifice, or a time-traveler's view of Asclepius at work?

The human body has long been considered a sacred and mysterious object: the physical manifestation of divinity, a hallowed vessel of God consciousness. We do not know what makes a body alive. We think we know when it is dead. But we have no definition of life. Is it any surprise then that surgery, the specialty that violently invades the temple of the soul remains a stronghold of myth, superstition and mystery? There is, even in this evidence-based world of modern medicine, an underlying uneasiness about what it is that surgeons do every day: the invasion of the confines of the human body, the subjugation of human consciousness, of spirit, that we take for granted, but not completely. It is just possible that we are overstepping our bounds as ordinary mortals, invading the territory of the gods.

There remains in modern surgery a mythology of surgeon as God, of procedure as sacrifice, of process as sacred ritual. What is most unclear is how we get away with it, if indeed we do. With no conscious concept of where the life force resides or of where the energy field begins and ends, we take a leap, as surgeons, into a completely uncharted territory. We skillfully fumble about with scalpels and scissors, clamps and retractors, never knowing if we are harming some unseen force that may affect our patient in unimagined ways for the rest of their lives. We rely on the cellular, humoral, mechanical repair processes of the physical body to return our patient to health. We plan for healed incisions and functioning physiology, wondering what other considerations of spirit, awareness, energy flow we have left unaddressed. Like any other ceremony, surgery is anticipated to proceed in a prescribed manner. When it does not, serious consequences are expected-- and I suspect, secretly welcomed. They confirm the necessity of preserving the ritual.

What is it about surgery that requires this almost sacramental ritualism? It may be because we still know so little about what happens during surgery: how anesthesia really works; what happens to consciousness and the soul while one is under anesthesia; why some do not awaken from anesthesia; why anyone heals from the trauma of the scalpel in the first place. Are there really energy fields about which we know nothing, but invade with every procedure? And who is to know when the unexpected and deadly will occur. Is it any wonder that we invoke superstition and prayer to improve our odds of success?

Surgeons are known, among their peers, as unusually superstitious practitioners. For scientists, they have a lot of irrational behaviors. Many will only operate wearing a favored piece of apparel, a scrub hat for instance, or carrying a special amulet. Some must always scrub at the same sink, open the soap in the same way, or scrub for precisely the same number of minutes. Some require a special music in their OR, a particular scrub nurse, a personal pair of scissors. Without these totems, they become anxious, irritable, or even violent. Though most would never admit their small acquiescence to the gods of healing, they are real, and they are considered essential to the outcome of surgery.

Surgeons all know of colleagues who are referred to quietly as "unlucky surgeons." There is almost a shunning of them. They are professional pariahs and rarely receive referrals of importance. Most practice alone, since no one wants to catch their unluckiness. It is perceived that something is wrong with them energetically, though I doubt that most surgeons would verbalize their feelings about those ill-fated colleagues in such terms. No matter how smart or technically proficient, they are not true High Priests in the surgical clergy. Like much of what happens in surgery, we don't know why these surgeons are so fated.

Omens are of particular significance to surgeons. A patient who feels certain they will die during surgery risks cancellation of their operation by a spooked surgeon or anesthesiologist. Wise surgeons listen carefully to their patient's wishes around surgery, believing on some level, that the patient has an uncommon insight into the future. Full moons are dreaded as portents of unusually violent surgical cases appearing in the ER. These actions suggest a degree of primitive spirituality reminiscent of witch doctors and voodoo, concepts that no modern surgeon would confess to honoring.

I am not suggesting that the unscientific behavior of surgeons is bad, or unnecessary. On the contrary, our rituals keep us on the side of the gods, the descendants of Asclepius, whose rod our societies proudly display. We bow to them and ask their assistance in every case that we do, whether consciously or not. Without them, we aren't really sure what would happen in that temple of surgery, the operating room.

As for me, if I need an operation, I'll make sure my surgeon is wearing her lucky scrub cap.

Healing Experiences In Rituals Of The Native American Church

Christian Dombrowe

Abstract

This qualitative, psychological investigation explores healing experiences of participants in rituals of the Native American Church/Peyote ceremonies. This study draws on interview data collected from nine participants of Peyote ceremonies. The co-researchers were five men and four women in the age range between their late twenties and early sixties. Five of the co-researchers were Euro-Americans, three Native Americans and one mixed Euro-Native American.

The data analysis resulted in the identification of seven core themes of the experience of healing in rituals of the Native American Church/Peyote ceremonies. These were: spiritual connection; enhanced self-esteem; emotional release, sense of community; physical recovery and support; insight and heightened awareness; and enhanced environmental sensitivity. By providing accurate accounts of healing experiences and in-depth portrayals of individual cases, this study aspires to contribute to a better understanding of the therapeutic potential of rituals of the Native American Church/Peyote ceremonies and the religious use of entheogens in general.

Research Participants

- Participants were selected based on the following considerations:
- Adult men and women who have been committed to the 'Peyote Road' (participation in rituals of the Native American Church as their primary spiritual practice) for more than a year.
- They have had a self-ascribed significant healing experience with peyote.
- They were willing to participate in the research project.
- The nine co-researchers that finally participated in the study were five men and four women in the age range between their late twenties and early sixties. Five of the co-researchers were Euro-Americans, three Native Americans and one mixed Euro-Native-American.

Procedures and Research Questions

Each interview lasted between one to three hours. A follow-up interview of approximately one hour was conducted with most of the co-researchers (some gave their feedback by email or telephone). The central research questions that guided the interview were:

What kind of healing effects do people experience in their lives through the use of peyote in a ceremonial context?

What kind of physical, emotional, mental or spiritual changes do people experience through their participation in peyote ceremonies?

THE SEVEN CORE THEMES

1. Spiritual Connection.

Participants in peyote ceremonies consistently report becoming aware of deeper spiritual reality within as well as around them. All of the co-researchers at one point or another in their many years of participation in peyote ceremonies experienced a relationship with a spiritual presence. This presence is sometimes recognized as their innermost identity and sometimes felt to be a greater power than their individual self or any worldly power. As a result of this the person's religious life is infused with a greater vitality expressed in intensified spiritual practice on a regular basis and a strengthened faith. For greater clarity I decided to divide the core theme 'Spiritual Connection' in three sub-themes. These are 'Spiritual Centering', 'Connection with the Sacred/Divine' and 'Strengthened Faith & Spiritual Practice'.

1.1 Spiritual centering:

Several co-researchers mentioned that an important part of their experience of healing in peyote ceremonies was to find their own spiritual center, to understand their own true nature and to be aligned with it. 'Spiritual centering' can be understood as the process of discovering one's essential nature, an unfolding awareness of one's spiritual identity beyond social roles and mental constructions.

Eating the medicine it strips you down to your core being. You realize that you are sitting down on the earth and there is the fire and so it brings you back to a natural state. Our normal state is not necessarily our natural state. So our normal state is to be judgmental, to be protective, to shield ourselves from people, just to always regard everyone as potential threat.... But the medicine brings you back to more of a natural state... that spiritual place is already there. You don't have to attain it; you just have to remove this blockage. (Interview #8)

1.2 Connection with the sacred:

A central aspect of the co-researchers' experience of healing in peyote ceremonies is their sense of coming into a direct relationship with a higher power, feeling in contact with a divine presence. Participants in peyote ceremonies are able to overcome alienation on a fundamental level. It could be described as "homecoming of the soul."

Love is the main element, the Creator's love. That is the healing power it has. Because through that, once you move into that place of love and compassion... that love is always there, it's never gone.... And that's what that medicine does. It removes that veil. That's why they call it medicine. (Interview #8)

1.3 Strengthened faith and spiritual practice:

As a result of discovering their spiritual identity and feeling connected to a higher power, the majority of co-researchers expressed that their spiritual faith and practice were strengthened. In this way the ceremonial experiences can be said to have a forming influence on participants' will, personality and character.

My experience in peyote ceremonies informs my daily life . . . [and that] has something to do with bringing the sacred into the ordinary. To look at my relationships as sacred. To look at my work as being the arena for the expression of my sacred nature. (Interview #1)

2. Enhanced self-esteem.

For many co-researchers a central element of their experience of healing facilitated through their participation in peyote ceremonies was to gain self-confidence, to feel an increase in their self-esteem. Singing in front of others, sharing oneself from the heart, expressing and disclosing one's inner life in front of others were central in this process.

So I feel like on an emotional-spiritual level that it gave me a new way to feel strengthened, a new way to feel strong about myself.... the Church really enhanced my self-esteem and really made me feel better about myself, made me feel like a strong human being . . . I used to think I was a terrible singer and I found my voice through peyote. And I realized that it was very sweet. So it was those songs that made me realize that I had a voice and taught me how to sing basically. So that was a big step for me, to be willing to do that and sing my heart out in the company of other people. (Interview #5)

3. Emotional release.

An important element of the experience of healing in peyote ceremonies is emotional catharsis (often is accompanied by physical purging as well). Defenses against experiencing one's emotional wounds become lowered. Through the dissolution of inner conflicts that were based on repressing parts of their emotional being, participants in peyote ceremonies come to deeper self-acceptance and self-love that is the basis for experiencing love and compassion for others.

[The peyote] has helped me realize things in my heart and release a lot of pain, emotional pain.... I remember one meeting... all of a sudden I found myself sobbing. It was really quiet. And I realized that I was sobbing, I was just uncontrollably sobbing, sobbing... it was just all this pain in my heart, about my father, and this horrible relationship, and all this dysfunction, all this pain, all this stuff that I was holding. And all of a sudden it was just releasing. (Interview #3)

4. Sense of community.

Several co-researchers stressed the important role of the circle in the experience of healing in peyote ceremonies. They mentioned feelings of love, unity and belonging in the circle, of being supported by a congregation of prayerful people, where everybody is treated equally with respect.

That's the beauty of the circle. The energy of the circle is that all the minds become one. The circle is what creates the healing.... We have to do our part too and that's connecting, allowing the openness of your heart and spirit, to be open enough to were it forms that connection with the other people, the love you feel for them, you know. And then around that circle it creates that healing energy. (Interview #4)

At the same time it was kind of overwhelming that feeling of love that reached everybody's heart... in the morning when the sun came up all felt it; we all felt something totally new. There was nothing in the way to express our love to one another and receive it too from nature and people. (Interview #6)

5. Physical recovery and support.

On the physical level the experience of healing in the context of peyote ceremonies involves cures of symptoms of various diseases. Not only infectious diseases were mentioned, but also alcohol and drug dependence.

I was trying to taper off drinking... I used that sacred smoke in that meeting.... More or less that's what I said: 'I am looking to you; I need your help right now. I don't need it next week or tomorrow, I need it right now, right here. Can you help me?' Like that and I put that smoke down. That's what I wanted. In the morning I felt better, somehow I just had a different outlook on life, on things, real happy, felt real good that peyote, full of peyote and I was wishing I feel like this all the time. It felt good, I wasn't high, just feeling good about life, appreciate people, appreciate my wife, you know. So I went back to my job. About four years, every day these guys would get off work and had that big tub full of beer. I walked past it, you know, it didn't bother me. When before I had been the first one over there. I just quit. (Interview #7)

6. Insight and heightened awareness.

The co-researchers consistently report increased mental clarity and a greater observational power of their consciousness. This affects not only their perception of the world around them–for example in form of an increased empathic connection to others–but as well their perception of their inner world. They become aware of previously unconscious attitudes and beliefs. Bringing these thoughts, beliefs and attitudes to the light of consciousness allows the participants in peyote ceremonies to move beyond denial, to come to a more truthful self-assessment. Some co-researchers also report receiving new knowledge that is communicated to them by the peyote, often described as emotional or embodied. Overall it can be said that the heightened awareness triggered by the peyote ceremony affects the participants' clarity of perception on all levels: somatic-emotional, mental, and spiritual.

I also have had the experience mentally of having realizations about a situation… that kind of insight has happened to me several times about different situations, like 'this is what's happening'. So I have got a lot of mental clarity…. Yeah, to me it makes me much more aware, makes me hear things more clear and see things more clear. Thoughts are clearer. (Interview #3)

7. Enhanced environmental sensitivity.

Co-researchers in peyote ceremonies report experiences of the sacredness of nature, of the immanence of the divine in nature, and of feelings of unity and communion with the natural world. They gain an understanding of the natural unity of Creation, that humanity is part of nature, and that Spirit is in all things. Consequently their attitude towards nature becomes more reverential, so that respecting and honoring the Earth is felt as a moral obligation.

I feel like being part of the Church, in the tepee, on the Earth, you know, with all that goes on in a meeting, has taught me respect for nature and respect for the Earth and the water and the importance of keeping these things clean and intact. And that is what we have to do for our children. So it really helped me to become aware of all that in a way that, once again I might have known on a certain intellectual level, but to make it part of my life in another way, and to really examine how each aspect of my life... impacts the seventh generation basically.... That is a result of my experience with peyote and the NAC. (Interview #5)

IMPLICATIONS OF RESEARCH RESULTS

The results in this current study contrast with experiential reports given by primarily white European or American scientists in the late nineteenth or early twentieth century. These individuals observed mostly psychopathological phenomena as a consequence of self-administering either peyote or the pure alkaloid mescaline (Anderson, 1996, pp. 79-105). This marked difference in reported experiences can be explained by environmental and cultural factors (Wallace, 1959). Whereas the predominantly fearful, negative responses that the majority of these early scientific explorers reported occurred in a non-religious setting without therapeutic intent, the co-researchers in the present study used the sacrament peyote in a serious religious ritual setting with healing intent. Certainly this observation is indicative of the importance of a mindful and reverential approach to the psycho-spiritual work with sacramental plant medicines.

The evidence of this study suggests that the therapeutic potential of peyote ceremonies transcends ethnic and cultural boundaries. As the co-researchers stories reveal, peyote ceremonies appear to affect non-native participants as well. Although the peyote ceremonies in the tradition of the NAC are a unique expression of Native American culture and identity, they have therapeutic potential and efficacy not only for Native participants but also for non-native participants.

Even though this research project has uncovered commonalities be-tween Euro-American and Native American participant's experiences, the research also revealed distinct features. For Native American partic-ipants the Peyote ceremonies tend to reaffirm their cultural identity and to strengthen their confidence in the validity of their cultural values and world-view. For Euro-American participants the Peyote ceremonies seem to facilitate a critical investigation of the world-view and values of their culture (recovery from an alienating materialistic, de-spiritualized world-view).

The testimonies of two co-researchers who were able to overcome their drug or alcohol addiction through the NAC ceremonies confirm the findings and observations of previous research on the healing potential of peyote ceremonies in the treatment of addiction. Yet the results indi-cate that the therapeutic potential of peyote ceremonies goes well beyond the treatment of addictive disorders, and includes holistic healing of the physical, mental, emotional and spiritual.

The co-researchers in the current study also reported greater mental clarity and ability to focus. Slotkin (1956) has pointed out that peyote teaches the participants in the ceremony through mystical experience or simply through a heightened sense of awareness. The co-researchers in this current study also reported gaining important insights into pressing life concerns that have therapeutic value. This matches findings of Soibel-man (1995) and Quinlan (2001) who reported that their co-researchers experienced profound insights as a result of participating in ayahuasca ceremonies.

The peyote ceremonies also offer participants profound spiritual heal-ing. The co-researchers in this current study reported gaining a new or renewed sense of connection with the sacred dimension of life larger than their ego identity They experienced an awakening to this divine presence. This finding corresponds with those of Soibelman (1995) and Quinlan (2001) who report that participants in ayahuasca ceremonies frequently experience direct contact with the divine. Together these findings suggest a unique potential of the ceremonial use of psychoactive plant sacraments in facilitating spiritual consciousness.

The current study also found that participants in peyote ceremonies experience an increased awareness of their connection to the natural world. Several co-researchers reported an increased environmental awareness and a more reverential attitude towards nature as a result of their participation in peyote ceremonies.

The customary view of peyote ceremonies as being solely a folk therapy for the treatment of alcoholism among the Native population has to be expanded. From the evidence of this and other research, the traditional ceremonial use of peyote is not only capable of inducing profoundly transformative and healing experiences, but also represents a genuine (and demanding!) spiritual practice. This spiritual discipline of ritual use of a sacramental plant medicine offers its adherents all the benefits one could hope to achieve from any other path of spiritual practice. This traditional ceremonial use of sacramental plant medicine involves the cultivation of concentration and mindfulness and the development of compassion, offers moral guidance for an ethical life, encourages the practice of selfless service, and contributes to the development of wisdom.

This research suggests a recognition and acknowledgement of sacramental plant medicine ceremonies. As practiced by many indigenous peoples and by an increasing number of Western adherents, they represent genuine religious traditions and spiritual practices in their own right, and they are a precious part of the collective cultural heritage of humanity.

Rituals of Transition and Transformation

Ralph Metzner

I PROPOSE THE FOLLOWING DEFINITION OF RITUAL: *Ritual is the purposive, conscious arrangement of a sequence of actions, at particular times and in particular places, according to specific intentions.* It can be seen that this is a very general definition – as "ritual" is indeed a very general and morally neutral concept. Whether a particular ritual activity is "good" or "bad", constructive or destructive, can only be evaluated by its outcomes or consequences, as "a tree is known by its fruits."

Rituals of Everyday Life

We are all familiar with the common little rituals that punctuate transition phases of our everyday existence. In the mornings we have the rituals of the toilet and of cleaning, shaving, dressing and perhaps exercising. At night time we have the bedtime rituals of putting on night-clothes, stories, prayers, good-night kisses. Parents with small children know how important it often is to the child that the exact same sequence of ritual elements is preserved, in order for the child to go to sleep peacefully.

The rituals associated with a family eating together are perhaps the oldest and most venerable in human life, going back to paleolithic times, when hominid hunters brought back meat from the hunt to share with the family and tribe. We also know the rituals of the family meal, and students of family life have pointed out how important family mealtime can be for strengthening the family bonds. Or how significant they can be in the development of neurotic disturbances, especially eating disorders, when food ingestion and sharing becomes laden with all kinds of extra emotional baggage, or the taking of food nourishment becomes a substitute for missing emotional nourishment. In such conditions, it's not so much the biochemistry of the food and drink that causes difficulties, but the rituals of the family meal that come overlaid with hidden neurotic or power agendas.

The consumption of our most popular psychoactive drugs, the depressant alcohol and the stimulant caffeine, is also surrounded by elaborate rituals, as we know well: the cocktail party, the college beer party, the conversations in the coffee house, or the ritual brewing of the morning "wake-up" cup. Researchers in the field of drug addiction have found that the typical addict is as dependent on the elaborate rituals of preparing for injection as he may be on the drug effect itself. Cigarette smokers know well the unconscious little rituals of taking the cigarette out of the packet, the lighting of the cigarette, for oneself or for others – all seem to be essential elements of the experience that soothes anxiety, overcomes withdrawal distress, and strengthens the habit.

The activities of flirting, mating, sexuality, love, courtship and marriage are all connected with numerous complex ritual behaviors, some prescribed by tradition, others suggested by glamorizing images in novels and films. Television serves up daily doses of ritualized sexual attraction, flirtation, seduction and courtship – often for sheer entertainment, but perhaps more often in the service of increasing sales of particular products through "brand awareness."

On the other hand, students of the Indian traditions of Tantra and of the Chinese Taoism have re-introduced ancient teachings of ritualized sacred sexuality into modern life again. In these traditions habitual sexual behavior can be transformed through intentional ritual to a spiritual practice in its own right. Mircea Eliade, in his work on Yoga, referred to Tantra as "ritualized physiology."

RITUALS IN ACADEMIA, RELIGION AND THE MILITARY

Ritualized behavior is pervasive in academic institutions, like a university. Typically, in collective ritual activities, there are clearly defined roles for different people to play. For instance, there is the ritual known as the "university lecture," in which one group of people, called "students," sit in a more or less receptive mode, listening to an individual called "professor" expounding on a selected topic. The two roles, speaker and audience, carry differing but reciprocal intentions that bring them together into the same setting, at the same time.

Human behavior in church, synagogue or temple is highly ritualized, so much so that for many people the word "ritual" is synonymous with "religious ritual." Religious rituals, it has often been pointed out, can become seemingly empty of meaning, just the mechanical repetition of certain words, phrases and gestures. What has happened here? It is when the original spirit or intention behind the religious ritual – which undoubtedly had something to do with connecting with divinity – is no longer alive for those who are leading the rituals, who are therefore unable to convey that spirit to the others. It is as if the ritual form, or ceremonial form, has been emptied of spirit – and people then feel bored or uninspired, not moved or uplifted. Some people seem to believe that all kinds of ritual are a good thing, and we need more of them in modern life. However, as can be seen in the example of religious ritual, the moral and social value of ritual is a function of the conscious intention behind the ritual.

Other areas of social life provide many dramatic examples of the moral neutrality of ritual *per se*. There are rituals of destruction and aggression – ranging all the way from the ritualized aggression of sports (and the associated spectator sports) like boxing and football; the fetishistic rituals of sado-masochism and bondage/domination in the sexual arena; the elaborately choreographed rituals of criminal investigation, policing, the judiciary and the court-room trial; and the alcohol-fueled hazing rituals of college fraternities. The dehumanizing training rituals of the military are also well-known: young soldiers are taught, in symbolic manoeuvers, how to immunize themselves against ordinary human impulses of decency and kindness, as well as neutralizing their conscience, in order to become more ruthless fighting robots. As is well-known, the Nazis were masters of ritual, using the power of uniformed masses of men, with torchlights, songs, marches and propaganda speeches, to accumulate and harness the human energy of zealous devotion to the party and the nation for their own in-group power agendas.

RITUALS IN MEDICINE AND PSYCHOTHERAPY

The ritual aspects of medical practice and psychotherapy are well-known and pervasive. The practice of medicine is not just the mechanical delivery of drugs or surgery. The way that treatment is presented, whether the physician regards his patient with respect or with condescension, the qualities of empathic support and human kindness – are all recognized (even if not always practiced) as essential elements of the treatment. Good medical training schools will emphasize the importance of a therapeutic "bedside manner" for successful therapeutic outcomes. The holistic medicine movement, in part inspired by Eastern medical traditions such as Chinese, Indian and Tibetan medicine, will consider all aspects of life-style, including diet, exercise, emotional stress, family dynamics and even astrological factors, as part of the overall picture of illness and recovery. These are all aspects of the time and space arrangements, the set and the setting of the interaction between physician and patient.

In the field of psychotherapy, the significance of the contextual ritual is also well appreciated. Psychoanalysis was sometimes called the "talking cure," but actually, in the writings of Sigmund Freud and his successors, the psychoanalytic healing ritual involved much more than talking. The psychoanalyst sits behind the patient, who is lying on a couch; the latter is instructed to consider the analyst a "blank screen" to which he can communicate his "free associations" -- free, that is, of the analysts potentially distracting appearance or verbal interpretations. One of Freud's most brilliant and innovative students, Wilhelm Reich, broke with that tradition and invented his own very different therapeutic ritual: facing the patient and observing the breathing movements of his body. He could connect those to psychic content, reading the pattern of muscular tensions he called the "character armor."

More generally, the importance of a warm, comfortable, safe, aesthetically pleasing setting, and empathic manner of the therapist is widely appreciated. These are all factors of ritual, believed to be and chosen to be conducive to positive therapeutic outcomes.

In all systems of healing, traditional, shamanic or contemporary, there are really two main kinds of intention or purpose that are incorporated into the practice – healing or problem solving, which involve dealing with the past; and seeking guidance or vision, which involve looking at the future. The parallel functions of divination in medicine are *diagnosis*, determining the root cause of the difficulty in the past, and *prognosis*, foreseeing the probable outcome of the illness in the future.

Western medicine and psychotherapy looks to the past for understanding the causal factors in illness or psychological difficulty: we ask where and how did the wounding, germ, microbe, virus, infection, or familial relationship difficulty begin? Shamanistic healers, for example in Central or South America, also recognize those causes of illness but are likely, in perhaps 50% of cases, to attribute the origin of both physical and psychic disorders to sorcery or hexing. Accurate causal diagnosis in both cases is recognized as being necessary to determining appropriate and effective treatment or cure.

Rites of Passage and Vision Quests

The seeking of guidance or a future vision for one's life was an essential core element of the passages of adolescence in traditional societies, especially among native North American Indians. The Plains Indians, such as the Sioux, would have their young boys spend several days on a vision quest in the mountains or wilderness, fasting and praying for a vision for their life. There would be extensive preparation beforehand and integration afterward by a tribal or familial elder. In recent years the practice of vision question or fasting alone in wilderness, seeking a vision, has been brought to many people at various transition points in their life, not only adolescence – but also transitions such as divorce, job changes, major deaths or losses in the family and so on. With such practices, one seeks to connect with inner sources of spiritual guidance, and healing through reconciliation with past conflict-laden relationships.

Rites of passage with a spiritual focus have for a long time been absent in the modern world. They've been preserved in attenuated and simplistic forms such as the rites of *confirmation* and *bar mitzvah* in religious communities, which for many adolescents don't carry much spiritual meaning anymore. Therefore, the re-introduction of *transition rites* or *rites of passage*, like the vision quest, into modern society represents a reconnection to the archaic life-wisdom practices of the ancient world and of indigenous societies, and as such presages the possibility of greatly deepened community and social cohesiveness and health.

DIVINATION RITUALS WITH AWARENESS AMPLIFIERS

Over the past thirty years I have been developing and teaching a set of ritual practices that I call *alchemical divination*, in which the focus is on psychospiritual transformation, described in the ancient symbolic language of alchemy, but also drawing on related practices of shamanism and yoga. These practices are rituals, in their formalized structure of question-and-answer processes, whether done as individuals or in groups. They can be equally applied to past issues and questions of healing, as well as future issues of seeking a vision or guidance for one's life. The steps of the ritual are purely internal, like a kind of meditation. But the question-and-answer format is similar to what one would expect to see with a physician or psychologist, or a diviner like a Tarot card reader or astrologer, where another person, with presumed unusual gifts or experience gives a diagnostic and prognostic "reading" of past causes and future prospects.

The advantage of having someone else providing the diagnostic and prognostic symbolic "signs" is that they are more detached and their perception presumably less distorted by the subjective wishes and fears of the seeker. However, the readings provided by such indirect divination tools ultimately will still have to be interpreted by the seeker. In the alchemical divination practices, the personal perceptual distortions of subjective wishes and fears are overcome (or at least reduced) by preceding and accompanying the question and answer divination process by practicing light-fire alchemical purification meditations.

The role of entheogenic substances (which have also been called psychedelic or hallucinogenic) in such divination ritual practices is neither necessary nor sufficient. Diagnostic and prognostic divination rituals can be done and are done in the ordinary waking state of consciousness and play a major role in all areas of life, including medicine and psychotherapy, as I've described above. The *entheogens act as non-specific perceptual awareness amplifiers*. What you become (more) aware of depends entirely on what it is you are looking at – the intention, purpose and context.

In other words, the therapeutic insights or creative or spiritual visions that may occur in such states are *not a drug effect*. The same drugs, taken in different contexts with different intentions – for example recreational, or even abusive, or with no conscious intention at all, will induce very different, widely divergent, non-useful, hap-hazardly irrelevant or even dangerous results – as a perusal of internet pages on these drugs will reveal.

If we compare how Western medicine and psychotherapy have incorporated psychedelic drugs into healing practice, with the shamanic healing ceremonies involving entheogenic plants or fungi, a perception of the importance of ritual is inescapable. Western psychiatric researchers investigating psychedelics as therapeutic adjuncts avoid the clinical coldness of a typical medical/psychiatric practice, instead providing a warm, comfortable setting with visual art and music, and the supportive guidance, as well as medical assistance if needed, of experienced clinicians for what can be a day-long experience.

The traditional shamanic or neo-shamanic ceremonial form involving hallucinogens like ayahuasca or psilocybe mushrooms or iboga, is a carefully structured experience, in which a small group of people come together with a respectful, spiritual attitude to share a profound inner journey of healing and transformation, facilitated by these powerful catalysts. A "journey" is the preferred metaphor in shamanistic societies for what we call an "altered state of consciousness." During the journey into the inner realms where the shaman seeks connection with spirits, the physical body is lying on the ground, protected from random or malicious intrusions by his/her assistants.

There are some significant differences between typical shamanic entheogenic ceremonies and the typical psychedelic psychotherapy. One is that the traditional shamanic ceremonies involve very little or no talking among the participants, except perhaps during the preparatory phase, or after the experience to clarify the teachings and visions received. The second distinctive feature of traditional ceremonies is that they are almost always done in darkness or low light – which facilitates the emergence of visions from inside. (The counterpart to that in psychedelic therapy is the practice of having the voyager wear eyeshades). An exception is the North American peyote ceremony, done around a fire (though also at night) – here participants may see visions as they stare into the fire.

The third distinctive feature of shamanic ceremonies with entheogens is that singing, especially the shaman's singing, is invariably considered essential to the success of the healing or divinatory process. Furthermore the singing typical in etheogenic rituals usually has a rhythmic pulse, similar to the fairly rapid beat in shamanic drumming journeys. Psychically, the rhythmic chanting, like the drum pulse, seems to provide support for moving through the flow or sequence of visions, and minimize the likelihood of getting stuck in frightening or seductive experiences.

In comparing Western psychoactive-assisted psychotherapy with indigenous entheogenic healing rituals, we can see that the role of an experienced guide or therapist is equally central in both, and the importance of set (intention) and setting is implicitly and explicitly recognized and articulated into the forms of the ritual. The underlying intention in both practices is healing and problem resolution. Interestingly, therapeutic results can and do occur with both approaches, though the underlying paradigms of illness and treatment are completely different.

The two elements in the indigenous shamanic traditions that pose the most direct and radical challenge to the accepted Western worldview are:

(1) the existence of *multiple worlds* or dimensions and (2) the role of *spirits* – beings normally invisible, though accessible in shamanic states of consciousness and practices, with whom one can communicate and who may offer assistance and guidance in the healing and visioning process. Of course, such conceptions are considered completely beyond the pale of both reason and science, though they are taken for granted in the worldview of traditional shamanistic societies – and by those Westerners, who through their own experience have liberated themselves from the thrall of preconceived materialist dogma.

It is worth mentioning that in the case of *ayahuasca*, there have grown in Brazil three distinct syncretic religious movements or churches, that incorporate the taking of ayahuasca into their religious ceremonies as the central sacrament. Here the intention of the ritual is not so much healing or therapeutic insight, as it is strengthening moral values and community bonds. The ceremonial forms here resemble much more the rituals of worship in a church, than they resemble either a psychotherapist's office, or a shamanic healing session.

There are also several different kinds of set-and-setting rituals using hallucinogens or entheogens in the modern West, ranging from the casual, recreational "tripping" of a few friends to "rave" events of hundreds or thousands, combining Ecstasy (MDMA) with the continuous rhythmic pulse of techno music. My own research has focused on what might be called neo-shamanic medicine circles, which represent a kind of hybrid of the psychotherapeutic and traditional shamanic approaches. In the past forty years or so I have been a participant-observer in hundreds of such circle rituals, in both Europe and North America. Entheogens used in these circle rituals have included psilocybe mushrooms, ayahuasca, LSD, mescaline, San Pedro cactus, peyote, iboga and others.

In these hybrid therapeutic-shamanic circle rituals certain basic elements from traditional shamanic healing ceremonies are usually, though not always, kept intact:

(1) There is usually at least one elder or guide of the ceremony, who handles the medicines, and who may speak or sing during the ceremony.

(2) Dedication of ritual space-time through the invocation of spirits

of four directions & elements, as well as other guiding spirits and deities.

(3) The structure of a rough circle is usually preferred, with participants either sitting or lying.

(4) An altar may be in the center of the circle, or at one side, where participants place personal objects of significance to them.

(5) Preference for low light, or semi-darkness; sometimes eye-shades are used; again, with exception of the peyote ceremonies, held around a fire.

(6) The use of music: there may be drumming, rattling or singing, by the conductor and/or by others; as well as evocative recorded music. Some groups, including the ayahuasca churches, also have periods of total silence.

(7) In general, the cultivation of a respectful, spiritual attitude, with conversational talk among individuals is minimized or totally excluded.

(8) Some variation of the *talking staff* or *singing staff* may be used in such ceremonies, in preparation beforehand and for integration afterwards. With this practice, which seems to have originated among the Indians of the Pacific Northwest, and is also more generally now referred to as *council,* only the person who has the circulating staff (or other object, like a shell or stone) sings or speaks, and there is no discussion, questioning or interpretation – a format beautifully designed to elicit profound sharing from the participants.

Experienced entheogenic explorers understand the importance of set and therefore devote considerable attention to clarifying their intentions with respect to healing and divination. They also understand the importance of setting and therefore devote considerable care to arranging a peaceful place and time, filled with natural beauty and free from outside distractions or interruptions.

Most of the participants in circles of this kind that I have observed were experienced in one or more psychospiritual practices, including shamanic drum journeying, Buddhist *vipassana* meditation, tantra yoga and holotropic breathwork and most have experienced and/or practiced various forms of psychotherapy and body-oriented therapy. The insights and learnings from these practices are woven by the participants into their work with the entheogenic medicines. Participants tend to confirm that the entheogenic plant medicines, when combined with meditative or therapeutic insight processes, function to amplify awareness and sensitize perception, particularly amplifying somatic, emotional and instinctual awareness.

In preparation for the circle ritual there is usually a sharing of intentions and purposes among the participants, as well as the practice of meditation, or sometimes solo time in nature, or expressive arts modalities, such as drawing, painting or journal work. After the circle ritual, sometimes the morning after, there is usually an integration practice of some kind, which may involve participants sharing something of the lessons learned and to be applied in their lives.

Selected References

Adamson, Sophia (ed.) *Through the Gateway of the Heart – Accounts of Experiences with MDMA and other Empathogenic Substances.* 2nd Edition. Petaluma, CA: Solarium Press, 2012.

Eliade, Mircea. *Yoga, Immortality and Freedom.* Princeton, NJ: Princeton University Press, 1972.

Fadiman, James. *The Psychedelic Explorer's Guide – Safe, Therapeutic and Sacred Journeys.* Rochester, VT: Park Street Press, 2011.

Feinstein, David & Mayo, Peg Elliott. *Rituals for Living and Dying.* HarperSanFrancisco, 1990.

Harner, Michael. *Cave and Cosmos – Shamanic Encounters with Another Reality.* Berkeley, CA: North Atlantic Books, 2013.

Metzner, Ralph. *The Expansion of Consciousness.* Berkely, CA: Green Earth Foundation & Regent Press, 2008.

Metzner, Ralph. *Alchemical Divination – Accessing Your Spiritual Intelligence for Healing and Guidance.* Berkeley, CA: Green Earth Foundation & Regent Press, 2009.

Metzner, Ralph. *MindSpace and TimeStream – Understanding and Navigating Your States of Consciousness.* Berkeley, CA: Green Earth Foundation & Regent Press, 2009.

Four Loose Stitches: Anomalous Healing Data and an Ouija Board Ritual

Stanley Krippner

The term "ritual" can be conceptualized as a prescribed, stylized, step-by-step, goal-directed performance of a mythological theme. It is "prescribed" by such practitioners as shamans, religious functionaries, or family or community elders. It is "stylized" in a form that symbolizes deeper meaning to the participants. It is "mythological" in the sense that myths are imaginative narratives concerning vital, existential human concerns, narratives that have behavioral consequences. It is "goal-directed" in that its performance is expected to lead to practical, observable results (Krippner, 2000).

Rituals are found in a variety of settings including children's games, life passages, institutionalized religious routines, obsessive-compulsive activities, and cultural practices. It is likely that ritualized behavior served an evolutionary function as part of a repertoire that detected and responded to external threats (Boyer & Lienard, in press).

Healing rituals are interventions founded on patterned interactions between clients and practitioners within the framework of a culturally shared belief system. Rituals maintain and improve the bond between

269

them and provide both with a conceptual framework that provides a sense of direction, mastery and self-worth. As a result, rituals help clients overcome despair and combat demoralization (Frank & Frank, 1990). The emotional intensity of rituals awakens confidence, hope, and a healing expectation, and thereby builds the morale that is necessary for staying engaged in the sometimes painful process of healing, rehabilitation, or personal change (Achterberg, Dombrowe, & Krippner, in press).

The Ouija board was first introduced to the American public as a parlor game in 1890. A typical Ouija board has the letters of the alphabet inscribed on it, along with such words as "yes," "no," "maybe," and "goodbye." A pointer of some type is manipulated by those using the board; someone (including the person or persons holding the pointer) asks a question and, for one reason or another, the pointer generally moves, stopping at certain letters or messages. These selections often spell out the answer to the question asked; at other times, the letters will produce gibberish.

THE RETURN OF MARILYN MONROE

While working at Maimonides Center in Brooklyn, I once joined a group of friends for an Ouija board session; they had been trying to contact the "spirit" of Marilyn Monroe, but without apparent success. Shortly after I joined the group, the Ouija board seemed to be providing answers to our questions. For example, when asked "How did you die?" the board responded "beautiful." The answer to the next question was "goodbye," and I commented that, like a sensible actress, Miss Monroe knew when to make a graceful exit.

Whatever the source of the answers provided by the Ouija board, its proper use demands a ritualistic approach. The session that I attended had started with the burning of a candle, the joining of hands, and a plea to the "spirits" to take the group's questions seriously. Following the departure of Marilyn Monroe's alleged "spirit," the group engaged in another ritual, thanking the "spirit" for her effort and holding hands again to complete the session. In my opinion, the use of ritual was an appropriate safeguard for those group members who were highly dissociative during much of the session.

The movement of the pointer often is attributed to invisible agencies such as "spirits," but most psychologists have concluded that those using the pointer are consciously or unconsciously selecting those letters that are being "read." When unconscious forces are at work, the user is often unaware of what is transpiring and may be engaged in "dissociation." I would define dissociation as reported experiences and observed behaviors that seem to have been partitioned from conscious awareness, behavioral repertoires, and/or self identity. These partitioned experiences and behaviors can be unconsciously directed to divert or to block streams of information from conscious awareness.

The movement of the Ouija board's pointer in the Marilyn Monroe session may have occurred while one or more members of the group was dissociating, allowing ideomotor effects to direct the pointer's movements. The term "ideomotor effects" refers to involuntary, unconscious motor behavior performed under the influence of suggestion or expectancy (Hyman, 1977). Hence, the Ouija board ritual can hardly be considered anomalous, but information yielded by this ritual sometimes is not easily explainable.

THE OUIJA BOARD FROM MAINE

The Ouija board had played a unique role in my life a few years before the Marilyn Monroe session. Even though I had complained of various symptoms, they had not been picked up by physicians during several annual physical examinations. Suddenly, I was hospitalized for internal bleeding in 1965. On the same day, Shirley Harrison, a "psychic sensitive» friend of mine from Maine, told her daughters she had to fly to New York City because «Dr. Krippner needs me.» Harrison added, «He is seriously ill with bleeding ulcers and will be operated on before Monday evening.» The operation for duodenal ulcers took place on Monday morning.

How did Ms. Harrison arrive at her diagnosis, a diagnosis that physicians had failed to detect despite my list of symptoms (abdominal pains, sudden weight loss, vomiting after meals, etc.)? Each night she consulted her Ouija board, asking her "spirit guides" to alert her regarding the well-being of her family and friends. When the Ouija board alerted her that someone was in danger, Ms. Harrison took immediate action. In this instance, she arrived in New York City, and spent the night praying for my welfare with a circle of my local friends.

However, my troubles were not over. The post-operative wound in my right side, left open to permit the drainage of waste fluids, did not close. Ms. Harrison visited me in the hospital, bringing her Ouija board along with her. It was a small-size version of the one I had seen earlier, but she did not want to alarm any hospital personnel who might enter my room at an inconvenient time. She was now so familiar with the process that she felt she did not need to employ a pointer. Her "spirit guides" communicated through the mini-board as she touched it, and her fingers rapidly moved around the letters and numbers as she verbally reported the message. I noticed that her words did not always match the letters that her fingers touched, and concluded that the Ouija board served as a "focusing device" for her, perhaps in the same way that I had observed a crystal ball or pendulum "focusing" the efforts of other "psychic sensitives."

Ms. Harrison told me that four stitches needed to emerge from the wound in my side before it would heal properly. Nevertheless, she continued, this would occur within three days. She gave me no information as to how these stitches would emerge, but expressed her confidence that my ordeal was nearing its end.

Nothing else had worked, so I took Ms. Harrison at her word, using mental imagery to evoke images of what she had termed "the loose stitches." On the second day of my attempts, two double-stitches emerged from the cavity, and on the following day the wound closed (Krippner & Welch, 1992, pp. 2-3). My surgeon was delighted and in a few days I was released from the hospital.

DIAGNOSIS IN A DREAM

There was one more round of anomalous information involved with my surgery. My physician had told me to avoid aspirin, because I was now quite allergic to the substance. Several years later, I was living and working in California but returned to the East coast from time to time, and still had a part-time position at Maimonides.

On one occasion, I returned for a lecture in Philadelphia and another in New York City. While in Philadelphia, I visited a walk-in clinic because I had developed a head cold. I had become accustomed to the sunny California climate and was not used to the chilly winters of the East coast.

The physician at the clinic told me that I did not have a fever and told me to buy a particular type of gum that would keep the cold in check. The name of the gum was "Asper-Gum" and I did not have enough sense to read the list of contents. If I had done so, I would have discovered that aspirin was the chief active ingredient.

The Asper-Gum worked well, and I went to bed in New York City thinking that I would be in good shape for my lecture the following day. In the middle of the night, I was awakened by a dream. In the dream, I was examining an X-ray of someone's stomach. The physicians agreed that it portrayed someone with a newly-developed ulcer. I awoke, wrote down the dream, and went back to sleep.

The next morning, upon visiting the bathroom, I noticed blood in my stools. I called a taxicab and checked myself into Maimonides Medical Center as an emergency patient. The same surgeon who had operated on me years ago was on duty and immediately ordered an X-ray. Indeed, an ulcer had developed—a small one, but one that would prevent me from delivering my lecture later that day. I was told that the entire audience offered prayers in my behalf, and my aborted presentation was published in the proceedings. The topic of the conference was unconventional healing (Krippner, 1978).

I spent three days at Maimonides, and the ulcer healed rapidly. I promised my surgeon never to take aspirin again in any form. Before I left the hospital, he told me, "I rarely recall my dreams, and I have never had a dream about you. But the night before you showed up in the emergency room, I had a dream that you had returned to Maimonides."

Reports such as this cannot be considered evidential. I had conducted enough research at Maimonides and elsewhere on anomalous dreams to know the role played by coincidence, faulty memory, and actual prevarication (Ullman & Krippner, 2002). But, for whatever reason, my surgeon's dream report coincided with my own dream, one that diagnosed the medical emergency.

My dream probably reflected my body's knowledge of its own condition, and there is some evidence that dreams often contain medical information (Smith, 2000). But if my surgeon's dream report was accurately reported, it was a remarkable coincidence, perhaps even an anomaly.

References

Achterberg, J., Dombrowe, C., & Krippner, S. (in press). The role of rituals in psychotherapy.

Boyer, P., & Lienard, P. (in press). Why ritualized behavior? Precaution systems and action parsing in developmental, pathological and cultural rituals. Behavioral and Brain Sciences.

Cardeña, E., Lynn, S.J., & Krippner, S. (2000). Anomalous experiences in perspective. In E. Cardeña, S.J. Lynn, & S. Krippner (Eds.), Varieties of anomalous experience: Examining the scientific evidence (pp. 3-21). Washington, DC: American Psychological Association.

Frank, J. D., & Frank, J. B. (1991). Persuasion and healing (3rd ed.). Baltimore: Johns Hopkins University Press.

Hyman, R. (1977). Cold reading: How to convince strangers that you know all about them. Zetetic, 1(2), 18-37.

Krippner, S. (1978). "Psychic healing"--A multidimensional view. In J. L. Fosshage & P. Olsen (Eds.), Healing: Implications for psychotherapy (pp. 48-83). New York: Human Sciences Press.

Krippner, S., & Welch, P. (1992). Spiritual dimensions of healing: From tribal shamanism to contemporary health care. New York: Irvington.

Krippner, S. (2000). Altered states of consciousness and shamanic healing. In R.

Heinze (Ed.), The nature and function of rituals: Fire from heaven (pp. 191-212). Westport, CT: Bergin & Garvey.

Smith, R.C. (1990). Traumatic dreams as an early warning of health problems. In S. Krippner (Ed.), Dreamtime and dreamwork: Decoding the language of the night (pp. 224-232). Los Angeles: Jeremy P. Tarcher/ Putnam.

Ullman, M., & Krippner, S., with Vaughan, A. (2002). Dream telepathy: Experiments in nocturnal extrasensory perception. Charlottesville, VA: Hampton Roads.

RE-MEMBERING HANDS: WILDERNESS RITES OF PASSAGE

DOMINIE CAPPADONNA

INTRODUCTION

OFTEN WE GO TO NATURE "AND LIE DOWN WHERE THE WOOD DRAKE rests in his beauty on the water and the great heron feeds"(1), and forget the cares of the world. We go to seek solace, to reach out for adventure and restoration, to find our church, our therapy office, and a place of comfort. The beauty and gentleness of the natural world can be soothing.

Yet at times a 'terrifying beauty' meets us where we expect to find solace. A jagged threatening rock blocking the way while climbing, a dizzying look over the side of a deep chasm. This jolts us awake, reminding us that our inner psyches and outside world are of the same texture. This jolt can help us to face what is difficult, by presenting a concrete experience of the dark aspects of existence on the hard ground of the earth, and the hard ground of our own psyches. Sometimes the body and mind scream as we release familiar creature comforts like resting in a flowered meadow, while our spirit rejoices in the freedom to explore outward-bound and inward-reaching realities that add texture.

Through our experiences of rituals and healing in wilderness, most often we come face to face with ourselves. We unearth what may be called our "secret undamaged self'" (2), our True Nature, our Essential Nature within; that which is open and vast, not torqued or influenced by what is arising in body, mind and emotions. In connection with our open radiant Being, we have an opportunity to reflect, rebuild, restore. Entering the more-than-human world of nature we may find restful restoration or frightening exposure to an environment that has become unfamiliar. In both are openings to the landscape of our own psyche.

Since we are not separate from, but a part of, the natural world by our very breath and birth, our self-perceptions can shift from ego-bound, to eco-identified awareness of the interconnection, "interbeing"(3), with all things. In Buddhist practice, for instance, we call this interdependence or Dependent Origination. Life experiences and spiritual practices can increase sensitivity to the more-than-human world.

Often, too often, in our culture, uninvited and enormously violent, collective events, such as Sandy Hook, Aurora Theater, Columbine, and 9/11 rip us open to a raw darkness that wrench our souls. Yet we have help. We have nature with whom to turn. We can heed the call of the wilderness. As we are meaning-making beings, our myths, rituals and practices found in Wilderness Rites of Passage Work invite us to explore our interior life. A call to integrate the darkest of the psyche's shadows, in both our daily life of self exploration and in the extraordinary times of collective tragic events. Healing rituals help us answer questions after a terrifying event and remember what can't be forgotten. What memories should we keep alive, and which should be allowed to fade? Which mental images give us hope? Which endanger our resilience? We know that memories can also serve as beacons of light on the long road to healing.

Wilderness Rites of Passage is a contemporary process to assist and celebrate an individual's passage from one stage of life to the next. The timeless universal transitions in life are birth to infancy to childhood to adulthood to old age to death. Within these universal stages are ones that evolved with the industrial and information age: adolescence, midlife, and living longer, all of which can evoke anxiety. An intuitive understanding of the stages from birth to death is rooted in the seasonal cycle from spring to winter. Thus, entering the more-than-human world of nature offers ease to the processing of life's transitions. Each passage between stages begins with a metaphoric death, a dying to the previous part of one's life. Wilderness Rites of Passage is, in a sense, a practice in dying and rebirthing. By heeding the Soul's call to grow, one learns to accept the little deaths along the way. We become more fully alive to the present, while preparing for the ultimate transition at the end of life.

Wilderness Rites of Passage assist individuals who are pushed out of balance by trauma of all kinds. Environmental and political crisis add tremendously to the disequilibria in these times and exacerbate personal stressors. As you will see in the account of our Wilderness Rites of Passage days after 9/11 in the Canyonlands of Utah, participants have a 'medicine bag' a template of rites and rituals. Rites support a loosening of attachment to one stage of life and to the traumas experienced so that one can die to the past and expand into the present. The rites present a balm to the soul's longing for wholeness, a time when the dismembered parts of one's being can reunite under the guidance of one's own True Nature.

Indigenous communities held and hold vital rituals to heal grief, terror, and trauma. Rites of passage, marking the developmental steps along life's path from birth to death, were crucial in creating a sense of security, continuity, and support. These rites were grounded in a perception of reality where essence shown through; where all things, animate and inanimate, carried soul, and thoughtful guidance met the urgency of each present moment. Our ancestors believed that all things are full of soul. They did not suffer the post-modern disorder of trying to seize soul and stuff it into egoic skins, as if the human body were the soul's and spirit's only house.

Over time, some of us who live in industrial growth societies have invested in cultural values that are less sustaining of our connections with one another and the earth. Yet, the pulse is right here to be reclaimed. We may experience a boundless connection with the world soul as a vital force pulsing in all things alive. This quickening energy is most easily sensed in moving tides, animals, birds, trees, each other, and our own breath. With practice, it is felt in mountains, boulders and earth itself. While we all have access to this primal source, how we interpret our experience will depend upon our worldview and our understanding of the nature of things.

Through a renewal of ancient and contemporary earth-based healing rituals and practices in nature, we can re-member the wisdom of our ancestors, renew our link with our own True Nature and recollect the soul of the world. Here we can begin to heal our personal and collective wounds as steps on the path forward.

As an eco-psychologist, I listen carefully to witness the realities of the human experience, encourage the resiliency of the human spirit, and seek the wisdom of the soul's dark journeys, all "as if your place in the world mattered"(4). Ecopsychology, formed from the Greek words, *eco, psyche, and logos,* suggests that we, in this multidisciplinary field, are interested in the soul of the home and the home of the soul. Thus, ecopsychology is concerned with the relationship between the human soul and the "soul of the world" (*Anima Mundi*) (5). In this way it might be said that it is the ecology of breathing awareness into our hearts and minds.

I proceed from the assumption that at its deepest level, the psyche/soul is bonded to the earth that mothered and fathered it into existence. John Seed, a rainforest activist , responding to a compliment that he was saving the rainforest, said, "I am part of the rainforest saving itself"(6). Conscious awareness of our interconnection offers us an expanded view of our belonging. Wilderness Rites of Passage can help us to practice this expanded sense of self and identification with all things.

Myths arose out of the first people's stories and chants in response to their own inquiry of life. To this day, myths as archetypal stories talk directly and powerfully to our inmost self. These can be understood literally as tales with recurring plots. But they are also symbolic, loaded with references to alchemical elements that resonate with essential aspects of all human psyches. This is readily seen when we remember a favorite fairy tale read to us by our parents. Upon recounting the tale to our children and grandchildren, we can perceive levels and depths of meaning that our ears are ready to hear.

The Wilderness Rites of Passage Journey:
Heeding the Call:

On September 14, 2001, with my co-guide we set out with twelve participants from 20-70 years old, who heeded their inner call. We arrive with emotions piqued; our fight, flight or freeze instincts acutely activated. The tangible tension of leaving our homes, so soon after the unexpected of 9/11, amplifies the state of agitation. Our intention is a sacred one: To attune with the Soul of the World, so that we can embrace wisdom and wound in the wild cradle of the natural world. We are guided by 'cairns', the metaphorical stone piles along a trail. These signify the developmental stages of the Hero's Journey as formulated by Joseph Campbell, the renowned writer on mythology and comparative religion.

Campbell suggests the Hero's Journey has three stages in rites of passage work: severance, threshold and re-incorporation (7). While Carol L. Flinders suggests a Heroine's Journey of three stages called: enclosure, metamorphosis and emergence (8). I see them as co-emergent, as dynamic and receptive principles. "A still point in the turning world"(9), in which men and women experience these interchangeably and/or as one, according to temperament. The active edge and quiet center help us find innate treasures to transform terror and brokenness. The gifts of rites of passage include insights and practical solutions to carry back into the world of family and community.

Arriving:

We arrive in the canyon lands of Utah raw with trauma. Met by the chaotic upheaval of a flash flood landscape gutted by a tumble of stone and severed roots, where once stood a spreading oak tree and grass. The scene mirrors the very rubble our weary eyes and hearts wish to escape. We scan the slice of sky that is visible through the narrow vice of canyon walls for contrails of passing jets. Are these routine flights, hijacked planes, or bombers carrying American's vengeance toward the ground of Afghanistan?

As I survey the canyon, my mind is pulled back to the New York City landscape where the World Trade Center towers had stood just days earlier. The graphic image of the severed hands of a flight attendant haunts me. I reflect on her, a woman combing her hair with capable hands as if to keep 'permanence' in place. By late morning her hands, bound, severed at the wrist, were found on top of a tall building close to the Twin Towers, dismembered as her plane exploded into the towers.

Each Wilderness Rite of Passage experience carries its own archetypal nuance. It is not surprising that the mythic image of the Handless Maiden archetype is pressing to the forefront of my mind; a journey from innocence, naiveté and ignorance to maturity and soulful wisdom. Joan Halifax describes the death that occurs in a shamanic initiation. "Death occurs in the process of dismemberment and sacrifice; the person is chopped up, tortured, and his or her bones are re-arranged"(10). On this quest, we are starting out emotionally ravished, and will seek a re-arranged wholeness.

Cairn One: Severance and Enclosure

Removal from our familiar world is a form of severance and bonding as a group is a form of enclosure. We begin by creating a base camp and forge a community. First few days are filled with teachings and tasks to prepare the group for their solo time in nature.

I am filled with images of severance that have set up house in my heart on 9/11 and will not leave. I share the tale of The Handless Maiden, paraphrased from the extraordinary telling of this story by Clarissa Pinkola Estes((11), around the campfire. The myth may provide a container for the wounds we bear and for the power of healing it fosters, perhaps clues used as breadcrumbs through the inner forest.

In brief, a poverty-stricken miller, makes a typically wretched bargain with the Devil. Unwittingly, he trades his innocent daughter for riches. Realizing the malicious deal the Devil has wrought, he is horrified, as he had not intended to sacrifice their precious child. When the Devil comes to claim the maiden, her purity prevents him from touching her. The Devil

281

orders the miller to cut off his daughter's hands, defiling her so that he can grab her. The miller does this, but the maiden remains so pure that the Devil cannot approach her. He leaves in frustration.

Her parents beg her to stay home so they can care for her. Yet the Handless Maiden, with her stumps bound in gauze, declines. She goes into wild nature, letting life take her as it might, and surrenders to the providence of All That Is.

She finds nourishment sipping on a pear, a food of the spirit, in the king's orchard. Seeing her unusual strengths, the king falls in love, and they marry. He has silver hands fashioned for her to wear. While she is pregnant, the king is called off to war. He leaves her under the loving care of his mother.

When the Handless Maiden gives birth to a healthy son, the king's mother sends a messenger to inform the king. The cunning Devil sees his chance for revenge. He intercepts the messenger and sends a message that she has given birth to a child who is half wild dog. The king, believing this, orders his mother to have the Handless Maiden and her savage child killed. To save their lives, the king's mother sends the queen and son away to take refuge in the deep forest. They find safety in a poor forest-dweller's inn. Over seven years, her hands grow back.

When the king returns from war, he learns of the Devil's treacherous deed. Grieving her loss, he searches for her for seven years. When he finds her she brings forth the silver hands she hid as proof of her identity. The king and queen, each changed and deepened, joyfully reunite. They return to their castle with their son and live happily and in peace.

We share haunting images of the severed hands, the violent loss of human life, and severing experiences of our own such as the loss of a child, parent or beloved. As well as severed by divorce, sexual or substance abuse, domestic violence, emotional imbalance, spiritual repression, disease and more. Commonalities lead us to bonding in this our enclosure phase. Instinctually, biophila -- humankind's positive connection with the living world -- calls us home in comfort, to "find our place in the family of things" (12).

CAIRN TWO THRESHOLD-METAMORPHOSIS:

Ceremony to deepen awareness, learn the ways of nature, and open our hearts and in preparation for four days and nights fasting and time alone in a solo site of one's choosing.

We offer soul-tending tools, shared safety parameters, teaching stories, sacred ceremony, and forays into the canyons to learn about natural resources. Taught how to find a power site for their solo quest: the active hunt to stalk and claim it, and the contemplative search to sit quietly and listen for the place to find the seeker. In ceremony, participants prepare for the liminal leap into the crack between the worlds, between the known and unknown, where metamorphosis and change takes place.

The night before leaving, around a roaring campfire, they release into the flames whatever stands in the way of a full commitment to walk through the portal into their solo experience. In its original meaning, threshold is the step-stone where the grain is flailed to release the kernel from the chaff. Metaphorically, threshold can represent an image of ego in service to the soul's mission (13). The solo time in nature is an opportunity for participants to embrace their authentic self.

We know that questions are common to the threshold stage. Questions rise like campfire sparks. "Will I die? Will wild animals eat me? Starve? Overwhelmed by loneliness, feel isolated and alone? Will I be able to encounter the turbulence within me? Will I be able to work with my fear? Will I be overcome by my emotions and by the past? Will nature speak to me? Will I act on the answers to problems? Will I fail? What if no answers come? What if I am bored and all this is a waste?"

I discover my own threshold, and ask myself, " How can I face my own darkness, my inner terrorist, my fear and deficiencies to gather the gifts of healing? What steps must I take to wake up and respond politically, socially and environmentally? I, too, will breathe, dream and slip into a metamorphosis on this journey, to find the work that awaits my hands.

At dawn, one by one, participants slip down the Rabbit Hole, the magical ceremonial passage that signifies their leave-taking and their invisibility to all but wild nature. They go out with a friendly hand. If the need arises, they have their buddies within the range of a loud whistle. We guides stand by at base camp. With them go their inspirations and promises to themselves to seek and find. Now, they go to the wild canyon in search of their own truth. The energy of the questers lingers on the morning breeze, echoing in the chirp of a Canyon Wren.

Cairn Three: Re-incorporation-Emergence

Four days later participants re-appear larger than life in silhouette against the morning sun. Out of red rock caves and from under cliff overhangs they come. Up clay paths, through sage, around thickets, and down river they trickle. They erupt from the mythological Rabbit Hole, grinning, weeping, silent and whooping, invigorated, weary, and inspired. All are deep with a pervasive stillness suggesting a stone has hit bottom in the quiet soul pool. As Wallace Stegner says, "wilderness is a part of the geography of hope"(14). Hope is a language of the soul. Participants return able to speak with the voice of the earth and the voice of their souls, "as if their place in the world mattered" (15).

Some come hand-in-hand their faces shining with victories over their own terrors. I reflect on the intimacy of reaching for another's hand in aloneness, fear and need. Re-membering on the brink of a ledge, those who leapt hand-in-hand from the burning Towers into the embrace of the ultimate threshold; the sacred necessity of other and the resilience of the human spirit.

Stories flow. Transformations reveal themselves through gestures, songs, dance, laughter, anguish, angry outbursts, words and hugs. The more-than-human earth has its way with us all. Emergence has its own rhythm; each person recounts varying degrees of metamorphosis, resolution and integrative insight.

"This is the first time I've faced my night terrors from my holocaust trauma. I stayed awake to them, courageously asking all the night creatures to bear witness. I fell asleep peacefully and slept for the first time in years."

"I felt my discontent and anger more strongly and the canyon was big

enough to hold me. I see my marriage is not."

"Within my circle of stones, I stood as an oak recalling my strength and perseverance in difficult earth activism activities. I saw I needed to bow more in gentle listening, as I had grown rigid and rooted. I saw flexibility in the bend of the willow."

"The song of the Canyon Wren awakened me to my innocence."

Large and small insights all have integrity and ring true as a bell. Between the group's stories, I share the story of a courageous friend of mine who held sacred ground during the Twin Tower destruction:

Avon Mattison of PATHWAYS TO PEACE awakens to the same dawn of 9/11 as the flight attendant who will soon lose her life and her hands. She is in the United Nations Building just blocks from the World Trade Center, preparing for meetings and to guide the delegates in the annual International Day of Peace on September 21st.

Feeling the assault of shockwaves from the explosions, she gathers other peace delegates in the Japanese garden in the inner courtyard of the UN Building. Clasping hands, they encircle the Peace Bell crafted from the melted coins of 60 nations and given to the UN by the Japanese in 1954. Holding hands, they pray for peace while terror spreads through the streets around them (16).

In the canyon morning, we find ourselves reflecting on the synchronicity of these powerful events, occurring on the same street, at the same time. The celebration of peace was not held that day, but the rehearsal and the fervent prayers of the delegates pave the way for the future end of war, in which we must all participate. The juxtaposition of the grossly unskillful means of the terrorist attack and the practiced meditations of peace delegates suggests to me the presence of light and shadow within every human heart. 'The path awaits our steps, the work awaits our hands, the world awaits our loving compassion." I envision the Handless Maiden's hands growing back while she lives in the heart of the wilderness. The restored wholeness created when the king and queen reunite, when the active and contemplative energies re-enter the world as one, bringing their offspring from the wild, symbolize hope for the world.

Conclusion: Beginning to Belong:

Like seeds bursting forth from fire, we a find terrifying beauty and awesome potential emerging from the experiences of wilderness rites of passage, the teachings of mythic imagination, and the horrors of September 11, 2001. This is a dark night of the ego, when the vast silence of the universe seems to shatter the fragile glass of the mind's noise. Parting clouds of smoke may reveal the naked pinnacle of truth that pierces our small skin to reveal our souls and the "Soul of the World." When we see that we cannot hold all mystery and power within our separate vessel of self, we grow our hands and reach forth mindfully, taking up our soul's gifts in service with the whole world. "When we love ourselves enough to listen with the ears of our heart to the other voices of ourselves speaking"(17), our soul rejoices to belong everywhere. Everywhere re-membered in this wild, beautiful, and suffering world.

1. Wendell Berry, "*The Peace of Wild Things*", *Collected Poems*, North Point Press, 1985
2. Terma Foundation, "*The Box Project*", 1995
3. Thich Nhat Han, "*Interbeing: Commentaries on the Tiep Hien Precepts*," Parallax Press, 1987
4. David Whyte, "*As if your place in the world mattered*", *River Flow: New and Selected Poems*, Many Rivers Press, 2007
5. John Davis, "*Home of the Soul, Soul of the Home*", Book Manuscript 2000
6. Joanna Macy & Molly Brown, "*Coming Back to Life: Practices to Reconnect our Lives, Our World*", New Society, 1998
7. Joseph Campbell, "*Hero with the Thousand Faces*", Pantheon Books, 1949
8. Carol. L. Flinders, "*At the Root of this Longing: Reconciling a Spiritual Hunger and a Feminist Thirst*", Harper-Collins, 1998
9. T.S. Elliot, "*The Four Quartets-Burnt Norton*," Harcourt, 1943
10. Joan Halifax, "*Shaman: The Wounded Healer*", Crossroads, 1982

11. Clarissa Pinkola Estes, *"La Selva Subterranea: Initiation into the Underground Forest", Women that Run with the Wolves",* Ballentine, 1992

12. Mary Oliver, *"Wild Geese": New and Selected Poems,* Harcourt Brace,2002

13. Terma Foundation, *"The Box Project",* 1995

14. Wallace Stegner, quote, Daily Camera, Boulder, CO, 2001

15. David Whyte, *"As if your place in the world mattered", River Flow: New and Selected Poems,* Many Rivers Press, 2007

16. Avon Mattison, Pathways to Peace, conversation 2001

17. Stephen Foster, Marion Little, School of Lost Borders, Conversation, 2001

Ritual, Prayer, and Healing

Lois Lighthart

One of the news magazines (*Time* or *Newsweek*) featured an article some years ago on the complete lack of ritual and/or ceremony in the lives of most modern-day Americans. This omission in our cultural mores leaves us, especially as teens, without a sense of grounding in, or connection to, the transcendent values that give meaning to human life. The article resonated with me, and I resolved to build on the nucleus of ritual which I already possessed, namely, the reading every morning of *The Daily Word*, published by the Unity School of Christianity in Missouri. My mother and I often listened to Bill Carlson, an announcer on KFAC Radio, Los Angeles, as he read *The Daily Word* every day at 8:45 A.M. (Those must have been summer mornings; otherwise I would have been attending classes at high school). We also subscribed to the booklet of the same name.

College came next . . . four years at Pomona, a Liberal Arts school founded by church people, albeit Congregationalists – not known for an emphasis on ritual or ceremony.

Then marriage, where for years, as a busy young wife and mother, a quick reading of *The Daily Word* was all I could manage in the way of a ritual. In later years, after having stumbled across the ideas of Carl Jung, and having also read the article mentioned above, I began to collect small objects which had some significance for me, and to place them on a low table which became my altar. I decided to light a candle each morning and to say a prayer affirming the unseen spirit and power which I believe underlie the material world. In addition to prayers provided by Unity publications, I began to write my own prayers. For example, with my candle lighted, I sit facing it, and say,

"Always coming from, yet resting in, that calm center point of light, love, and peace which is my only true self, I express that self serenely, with God as my source of health, strength, and ideas. It is a paradox that in doing this I do not deny, resist, nor look away from that vast and dark matrix of chaos and shadow which is an essential part of life, and therefore of me, and out of which order, value, holiness, and joy, are somehow mysteriously born. Hestia, Hermes, Hephaestus and Christ, be with me in spirit; the four directional angels, Uriel, Gabriel, Raphael, and Michael, and my guardian angel (who has a name but it's my secret*). Amen"* (Extinguish candle)

I close my morning ritual standing, facing eastward, asking this blessing,

"The light of God surrounds me; God is with me, and in me."

Then I ask a personal blessing for each member of my earthly family, and for any close friends facing a special challenge. As I hold each one in thought, I picture them in their approximate physical location, and, turning that way, extend my arms upward, saying:

"The light of God surrounds you; God is with you, and in you." (This is an abbreviated version of my favorite Unity prayer: *"The Light of God surrounds me (you); the Love of God enfolds me (you); the Power of God protects me (you); the Presence of God watches over me (you); wherever I am (you are), God is."*)

Another of my original prayers came about as an attempt to provide myself with an alternative to The Lord's Prayer which more closely reflects my personal beliefs. It goes like this:

"Praise and thanks, Great Father and Great Mother of the universe, together one life force. We acknowledge and honor You, living in our bodies, minds, and hearts, as well as in the wider world, and affirm that from your holy union within us, the Divine Child is continually reborn, inspiring us to live creatively, helping us find daily what is ours to do, the strength and will to do it, and the grace to do it graciously. Knowing Your forgiving love

for us, we can forgive ourselves and one another, and keep You alive in us, expressing through us, forever. Amen"

A separate prayer to honor the neglected Feminine, inspired by the reading of Jean Shinoda Bolen's **Goddesses in Every Woman**, goes:

"Hail! Queen of the Night, and Goddess of the Day! I acknowledge with loving praise the feminine half of life as expressed and represented by all the goddesses, wherever their spirits reside, within and without . . . the ancient ones: Gaia, Isis, Ishtar-Astarte-Innana, the Greeks: Aphrodite, Artemis, Demeter, Hera, Hestia, and Persephone; Norse Freya, and even Kali. To all of them I say, 'Thank you for your constant presence, and readiness to lend you strengths and inspiration to any task or challenge.' Strong, capable, and creative women through history, teach me, inspire me!"

Yet another that I made up addresses the three transcendent entities I prefer over "Father, Son, and Holy Ghost", and which encompasses some of the Jungian concepts I learned, thus:

"Goddess, God, and spirit of Christ, my Trinity: Bless my mind with focus and vigor, my body with radiant good health, my soul with inspiration, and my heart with love. Bless me with awareness of the Shadow, both personal and collective, and recognition of other inner figures and their significance. Keep me ever mindful of Trickster and ways to honor him, awaken my positive animus men – may they wax stronger than their negative counterparts. Help me to better know the goddesses within, especially Hestia and her sacred hearth, from which I obtain warmth and light, and from which I go forth to greater expression of the Divine Self within me, always keeping wholeness, not perfection, as the image to grow toward. Thank You!"

These creative efforts to put into words my evolving spiritual life, as well as three years of work with a Jungian analyst, have proved to be healing over time in several ways. Nervousness, anxiety and depression have been psychological burdens during my entire adult life, and I am increasingly able to deal with them constructively. One reason that Prayer has become a mainstay for me is that I really do believe in its power, not just as an inner comfort, but as an agent of change in the world. In 1988 I wrote the following essay that expresses this belief.

PRAYER POWER

Prayer, to me, is what occurs when human thought, prompted by love (sometimes accompanied by fear), reaches out to the creative power of the universe in an effort to bring some condition more into line with what one senses to be a higher and better expression of life. The problems of the world today are so enormous, so complex, and (thanks to communication technology and the ever-zealous media) so continuous to our attention, that it is easy to feel overwhelmed and immobilized. What can one person possibly do that will make a positive difference in the face of the many crises before us? If «You Can›t fight City Hall!" as the old cliché goes, who can possibly feel up to taking on Big Government, the hegemony of corporations, the Military-Industrial Complex or international terrorism, not to mention the growing numbers of homeless, the tides of Third World have-nots, recurring racial strife, AIDS, environmental deterioration, and on and on!

Feelings of hopelessness and powerlessness are surely among the most frustrating and debilitating of human emotions. They leave us weak, vulnerable to depression and other physical and psychic ills. Is there really nothing one can do? Don›t believe it! There is always prayer. And prayer does make a difference -- always! Though I may not see the specifics which I hold in mind come to pass, a difference is always made on the side of Good. This I believe. Is it just wishful thinking? I don›t think so, and my reasons for believing so are rooted in the following argument.

The most striking fact that's come my way in many years is contained in this excerpt from a commencement address made in June, 1981, at the University of Chicago by astronomer/physicist, David Schramm. (Ref: Christian Science Monitor, June 17, 1981, pp 12). He said, in part, (italics are mine): "...in particular, the developments out at Fermi Lab and other major particle physics centers have shown us that matter is not just the three elementary particles we remember from high school (neutron, proton, electron) but that the neutron and proton are made up of three quarks each, and these quarks seem to be true point like particles that do not take up any space at all. We are now reaching the view where matter is completely empty, with the mass being contained in points that occupy no space, and the only things that give matter is size, shape and dimensions are the *forces between the points.*"

Those «forces between the points» must be some forces! Everything that we see and touch, hear, smell, or taste, depends on these powerful and unfailing forces. Poet Walt Whitman wrote years ago of the «body electric.» His intuition was beyond the scientific knowledge of his day. Forty years ago in a college physics class, I was incredulous when assured that apparently solid objects were, in fact, mostly empty space. Now, if I understand Mr. Schram correctly, it turns out they are entirely empty space!

Christian Science founder Mary Baker Eddy was on target when she declared «All is Spirit.» She, however, looked upon Matter as something opposed to, separate, and different from Spirit, whereas it seems to me that so-called «matter», its solidity being totally illusory, is more akin to spirit than it is different from it. Apparently, there is no identifiable matter in Matter.

This concept opens the door to a new understanding, for me at least, of how the changes called «healing» and «miracles» are wrought by faith and prayer. Those «forces between the points» must be a very basic energy, akin, if not identical, to electricity or magnetic force. I believe that two other forms of energy, (hitherto unrecognized as such by traditional science), are Love and Thought. I further believe that love energy and thought energy can be superior in power to those wonderful, dependable forces which hold the physical world together and give all things their unique qualities.

Love, (that mysterious phenomenon that flows between humans and gives meaning to life, and flows as well from God to the created universe and from humans to God), and Thought (those prodigious creative mental powers unique to humankind) -- can they not be accepted as kinds of energy, different from, but possibly superior in power to those operating on the physical plane? And, what is prayer but these two forms of spiritual energy -- Love, and Thought -- combined to achieve the ultimate in power. Human thought, prompted by love, reaching out to the creative forces of the universe -- God, if you will -- in an effort to bring about a change in conditions more in keeping with what we sense life could be, is meant to be.

Believing these things about prayer and its power, I can give up for all time the thought that I am, or ever could be, helpless, hopeless, or powerless. For no matter in what condition of illness or crisis I might find myself, my loved ones, indeed, the planet itself, I can always remember to affirm my spiritual self and the spiritual basis of the world. I can always think a positive thought, can always love and appreciate something or someone, and thereby find an inner peace, knowing that the energy I generate in so doing goes forth to cause good results, somewhere and somehow.

Finding Home: Celebrating Sacred Space

Marcie Telander

Happiness…not in another place but this place, not for another hour but for this *hour*.   --Walt Whitman

I WAS MEANT TO BE HERE, IN A CABIN BY A RUSHING MOUNTAIN STREAM, 9,000 feet up in the Colorado Rockies. I have discovered that home is not based on the people, but the natural environment that surrounds me, and the spirits which dwell there. And when you marry a place that loves you back, the right tribe and the true family will always gather.

But life certainly wasn't this clear or simple for me several decades ago. After living nine demanding and spirit-straining years in Chicago, I realized that I was constantly "passing the communion", giving the holy bread to someone who needed it more. I was busy being an advocate for the speechless and oppressed, stage-managing and guiding others' emotional growth. I was dedicated to bringing expressive arts programs to inner city homeless, gang members, runaways and battered women. I was traveling to Indian reservations and communities around the country whose natural environment had been raped and abandoned by large mining and lumbering industries. I wished to honor their roots and struggles and the organic ways they expressed the stories of their own personal transformation.

Then slowly, as so often happens, I became ill, chronically exhausted-- never really sick, never really well. I was losing myself in the murky realm of "just existing." I was suffering from compassion fatigue, and eventually recognized the physical depression that precedes a spiritual crisis.

I was a zealous missionary who desperately needed to learn what she had been professing to others. I badly needed to find home, both within and outside of myself. While visiting friends in a remote part of Colorado's Western Slope, I was struck with love. The moment I rounded a big bend in the two-lane leading to Crested Butte, I knew I had come home. The tiny village nestled into the bosom of a mountain named the Red Lady, encircled by the powerful and feminine Elk Mountain range. I wanted to turn myself over to the sacred geography—the *genius loci* and spirit of the place. This was God's country and the Goddess' valley—all the extended family I needed. It took my partner, Mark, two cats, and me just two weeks to move lock, stock, barrel to the cabin in the valley by the river. This has been our home for 29 years. It wasn't easy but it has been worth it—proving that impulsive, impractical and financially impossible acts can also be life-saving rites of passage.

I had learned a great deal in my travels from native medicine people and healers. Now it was time to bring out the tools in my spiritual medicine bag and tend to myself. The wisdom of my body's demand that I physically slow down and conserve energy was a true blessing. I was invited to look at the universal in the unique, to sit in the sun next to the cleansing river in our back yard, and to appreciate the microcosm of my own garden. I walked and walked. I couldn't climb every mountain, but I discovered that a gentle hike garnered as much guidance and information. Every time I set out into the forest, I recognized I was beckoning synchronicity. In these walking meditations I was seeking and receiving "mini" vision quests. The "A-ha"s and "Amen"s were constant. With the noise tuned down, I made room to deeply experience the seasonal rites of passage, both internal and external, that nature makes available in every moment.

In a gentle way, I simply went wild. I stopped questioning, reasoning, and getting stuck with analysis paralysis. I entered Nature on her own terms and tried to follow her commandments.

Ritual will have its way with us, and we do well to honor its requirements. I learned that every ritual, no matter how formal or informal, requires seven stages. I have found it helpful to identify the seven stages through alliterations: purpose, preparation, purging, patience, playfulness, presence and promise.

I knew I had come to the Elk Mountains with a <u>purpose</u>—it was very simple: I was lost and losing my health, and I wanted to dwell and heal. I realized that I wasn't really being impulsive. The <u>preparation</u> for this part of my faith-walk had been in creation for over a decade. I had taxed and over-extended myself to the point of crisis, so no more preparation was necessary. The ritualized <u>purging</u> was implicit in the process of scaling down my entire life gatherings into one small, six-by-ten-foot wooden trailer.

<u>Patience</u> was one of the most difficult parts of the ritual for me. Living in a cabin in an ecosystem with eight months of snow, and a required familiarity with 19th Century frontier existence, truly challenged me. We experienced faulty leach-fields, plagues of voles, mice and bats, five feet of snow, frozen pipes, a flood, drought, break-in bears, snowbound and housebound weeks, a 125-foot tree falling on our cabin, and the threat of a highly-toxic molybdenum mine digging in next door. Challenges to patience included not only in the robust requirements of high altitude life, but also -- in the depressed ski-town economy – taking low-paying, seasonal and part-time jobs. Somehow we made it work. .

For <u>playfulness</u>, we learned to value entertainment that was simple and inexpensive. We celebrated rain falling on the tin roof in the spring, the return of the hummingbirds on May Day, and the first and last snows of our eight-month winters. Spontaneous rituals grew out of everyday necessities. When the plumbing didn't work we built a sweat lodge, then after the sacred Inipi ceremony, we bathed in the local warm springs amidst gently falling snow. Our social life was equally rich. We sat out under the stars with friends watching meteor showers and spectacular comets, or played classical music on the deck for the elk herds who paused to listen as they made their way to winter pastures.

Most importantly, I learned self-acceptance. Unlike many of the local

Crested Butte villagers I am not a backcountry skier or a marathon biker. I do not climb "Fourteeners", the rugged mountain peaks of 14,000 feet or above which surround our valley. I move slowly, listen closely, and give myself much time to simply *dwell*.

I learned that there is a sacred presence available to guide and teach us, if only we will listen closely and celebrate its mysterious voice in our "everyday" spontaneous rituals. I began to accept the promise: that the river flows by my door, and that living with conscious simplicity would always provide balm for my depleted spirit.

The rite of passage of coming home taught me: you can only, truly become creative when you recognize and honor your limitations. Through the teachings of this still, quiet voice that inhabited the daily "spontaneous vision quests", I changed my existence. Instead of traveling long distances to serve others, I developed a rich private psychotherapy and phone consultation practice with people around the country.

The message was exquisitely simple—stay rooted in your own landscape.

What this meant was that partner Mark and I agreed to marry our small, one-acre environment. It meant a dedication to what Scandinavians, Europeans, and recently Americans, have termed "deep ecology." This is the life devotion to support, conserve and advocate for one single, naturally-occurring watershed.

This would be our lifetime commitment to honoring and preserving *Home*. What this did not mean was to isolate or become environmental elitists. Thus, for almost a decade we listened intently to the presence and the promises of the small island of our land, an unexpected "wet dream" in the middle of the dry and drought-wracked West. This unusual mountain island is bisected by a series of springs and the swiftly flowing East River, which delineates our "backyard."

We did not move a stone, or plant a flower for eight years. We sat, asked, and were guided. We learned from local Ute Indian medicine people that our cabin is situated on the site of sacred land called the *Pahvant*, or "healing waters." This land, at the confluence of many watersheds, including our three tributaries, constitutes a powerful sanctuary. It was here that the Utes traditionally gathered, shared ceremony and rites of passage, and agreed to leave conflict outside of the fecund circle where they camped each year. When we had watched and listened long enough to both inner and outer nature, we began to make the little wise acre we steward a place for sharing many kinds of celebrations. We wanted others to share the transformative quality of sanctuary that our home place has made available to us.

For 25 years, women's, men's and family celebration groups have met here. We continue to celebrate births, baptisms, marriages, hand-fastings, coming of age rituals for adolescents, and cronings (or coming-of-age-again) for women moving into their 50's and 60's. We have held blessing and releasing memorials for two-legged and four-legged friends who have passed on. We have witnessed the closure of relationships which have finished their natural course, as partners honor the formal separation of their paths.

Celebrations of the seasonal festivals of the year, including full moons, solstices and equinoxes, are honored in the sacred saunas that we share with ongoing ritual groups. Being Swedish, it was a priority for me to build a wood-burning "wet" sauna for both physical and spiritual detoxification. In recent discoveries archeologists and pictographers believe they have found proof that ancient Scandinavian explorers brought the purging ritual of the sacred sauna to North American Indians. In fact, it appears that both the Inipi and the sacred sauna share some similar language, such as "loylie," which can be translated from both Swedish and several Plains Indian dialects as "the spirits come." We enter the purgative womb of the sauna the same way Native Americans enter a sweat lodge: with reverence for the expectation of the presence of Spirit and the guiding promise which awaits us here. We celebrate the four sacred directions with four rounds of sweating, chanting and praying. Leaving the sauna, "new-born and salted" we jump off the deck and into the snow-melt waters of the East River. Purged and regenerated, we share a potluck and our sauna visions around an outdoor council fire.

After years of tending, our garden and yard have been designated a "Backyard Wildlife Habitat" by the National Wildlife Federation. Every summer we host local children's adventure and ecology camps. The Crest-ed Butte International Wildflower Festival brings many participants here to Wetlands Conservation workshops and biodynamic gardening tours. I host several retreats during this festival in which adults are urged to become kids again, and build secret forts and fairy houses all around the garden. Writing retreats, storytelling concerts, poetry and music perfor-mances are held here throughout the year. At our Autumn Equinox gath-erings community members of all ages come together to create large effi-gies, aspen leaf and wildflower wreathes and costumes for one of Crested Butte's most beloved traditions. This is the celebration of "Vinotok," our Fall Harvest and Medieval Festival. I created this all-community festival 23 years ago, to celebrate our Old-Timers, featur.ng the personal stories of the miners and ranchers of all ethnic backgrounds who homesteaded this valley.

Vinotok is a Slovenian word that, loosely translated means "the season when the grape harvests are brought in and wine is made." It reminds us of the Slavic background of many of our valley's founders and culture-bear-ers. It also celebrates a long-time Crested Butte tradition in which the Slavs, the Italians, and the Scotch-Irish emigrants would compete each fall to see who had put up the very best homemade wine. We continue the old country ethnic traditions of wine tastings, all-night lamb roast, polka dancing in the streets, and the burning of a large effigy.

Included in this autumnal September event are evenings of storytell-ing around a roaring fire and ancient circle dancing by harvest lads and lasses crowned in fresh flowers and wearing medieval attire. These events are led by the Harvest Mother, played each year by a very pregnant local woman who represents the bounties of Mother Earth. A great procession, which moves down the main street of the village, performs the story of the Harvest Mother and her consort, the Green Man who is the symbol of irrepressible joy and fertility and the masculine protector of all creatures and growing things. The Great Grump, a giant effigy made by local chil-dren and a blacksmith artist, is carried majestically through the streets. The wild-looking effigy has been filled with "grumps" or pieces of paper upon which community members write the things they would like to release and banish from the passing year. These will be burned with the Great Grump in a three-story bonfire at the crossroads of the town.

The ancient, transformative ritual of banishing the past and beckoning blessings from the future are alive in this homecoming and harvest celebration turned forward. The sculptural metal and paper effigy of the Great Grump is now the scapegoat, bearing the burden of that which we wish to purge from our lives. As the huge bonfire burns against the night sky, we give thanks that our requests for guidance are being carried upward to whatever nature spirits oversee the new seasonal change of winter. This celebration of the great Feminine and Masculine is filled with singing, drumming and dancing long into the night around the giant bonfire. It is joyous, youthful and lusty, reminding us that the introverted, contemplative energy of eight months of snow will soon be upon us. The celebration is age-free, or as the local saying goes, "during Vinotok, every woman becomes a maiden and every man is a Green Man!" Each year the many skiers and snowboarders who live in Crested Butte believe that taking part in the bonfire ritual will assure them of luck, speed and safety during the coming winter. In a community of 3,000 full-time residents, it is meaningful to see all of your neighbors gathered around the Vinotok fire. This reminds us that the months of cold and snow are very near and that the most important harvest of our isolated mountain community is the abundance of shared personal stories and a communal generosity of spirit.

For me, the creation and sharing of this Autumn Equinox celebration with my extended family is the dream of a lifetime—one that continues to come true year after year. When one commits to the spirit of a place and is willing to see the sacred in the everyday, endless opportunities for transformational events present themselves. Not only do spontaneous vision quests appear in our mundane lives, we can be guided and directed to animate large ritual festivals such as the Vinotok Harvest Celebration.

Large or small, there is no difference between the promise and guidance potentially available in ritual. We can change our lives on a very personal or a group level. If we remain in a state of awareness, we are already prepared for the "immediate apprehension of the Mystery." The only differences I now perceive between spontaneous vision quests and the carefully designed rite of passage are in the amount of time spent planning and the witnessing of the event by others.

Does a woman have to make a geographical change to find her center and reclaim her life? No. But something major in her consciousness must move to higher, healthier ground. The word *karma* in Sanskrit simply means "action." That is what assists us in turning a dwelling into a home.

By allowing ourselves quiet time, walks in nature, prayer or meditation, we can be in communication and deep relationship with a loving energy that both nourishes and spiritually informs us. I learned to seek out and welcome what I call the spontaneous vision quest, the sacred in the seemingly small and ordinary. To sacralize our everyday reality is to be open to the mighty in the minutia. To live consciously within the seven steps of ritual invites and recognizes spontaneous vision quests, which over time transform our lives. This is the way of "godspeed", of the slow sacred. It is not the sudden thundering epiphany, or received knowledge that "slays one in the faith", or the all-knowing-forevermore answer. This is the divine manifested in daily-ness.

These natural moments of recognition and transformation align directly with each human's spark of unique spiritual *genius*, the still quiet voice of intuition. This truth-seeking and truth-revealing inner voice recognizes the larger Voice that is calling each of us. For me, living in a sacred manner has meant attempting to in-dwell in one watershed, one small acre of land, so intently that no bid for attention will pass by. But if we follow that truth-revealing Voice, we will find that place-- our true spiritual home-- wherever we are.

Surround Me

By Marcie Telander

Surround me
with the aftermath of love;
share our elixir,
toast the final draught that cures, heals.

Gather it by the door—
captured in rain barrels or
pumped from loss' own deep well.

Clear, clean and un-adorn walls—
hand scrub floorboards
throw wide windows.
Then, let us two make our bed,
heads bending together
over handwoven sheets, soft old
blankets and room for the dog and cat.

Make our house a closure to all sorrows,
for to believe this world
is home
is a traveler's most
voluptuous dream.

May the Gods Be Present: Depth Psychology Therapy as Ritual

Chris Downing

HONORING THE SACRED AND NUMINOUS DIMENSION OF THERAPY MEANS inviting in the gods and goddesses associated with *liminality*, with the crossing of the border between the profane and the sacred, between up-perworld and lower world. It means attending to how Hades and Perse-phone, Hekate and Hermes, Asklepius and Dionysos, Athene and Aphro-dite make their presence felt in the consulting room.

It is easy to discern in the consulting room the lineaments typical of the ritual pattern: separation from the profane world, initiation into a radically different, transformative, sacred realm, and return to the profane world in some way changed. The therapy hour is like the central moment in initiation rituals; the rules of the everyday world are suspended and we are encouraged to re-enter (wakingly) into dream-making, myth-making, consciousness.

The focus on the liminal, on the crossing of the border between con-sciousness and the unconscious is what makes depth psychology depth-full, makes it a psychology dedicated to the soul not the ego, an imaginal not a cognitive psychology. Depth psychology seeks to help us toward the depth dimension of experience, into what mythologies call the "underworld" and thus into a sacred realm and engagement with gods and goddesses.

In therapy we enter that realm willingly, out of a longing for depth, soul, transformation. Nonetheless we often find entering that realm terrifying; we often feel ourselves subjected to an abduction. I think of Inanna naively preparing herself for a visit to her just-widowed sister, Ereshkilgal, goddess of the Sumerian Land of No Return, adorning herself with all her *me*, all her emblems of upperworld power—as though one could go to the underworld like a tourist visiting an exotic land. But gate by gate, her me(s) are taken from her; by the time she arrives she has been stripped naked. Greeted by her sister with the eye of death, she is turned into a piece of rotting flesh hanging from a hook on the wall. I think of Persephone, reaching for the beautiful Narcissus that seems to promise something new, and finding herself seized by the dark god of Hades and torn from all she has known. I also think of Jung, after his break with Freud deliberately going after the myth that was living him, but then discovering himself in the midst of a psychotic-like process that might well have destroyed him. We know how it all turned out (just as we know that Abraham did not have to sacrifice Isaac after all), but none of them-- Innana, Persephone, Abraham, or Jung—knew that at the time.

This becomes painfully obvious if we allow ourselves to read the "Confrontation with the Unconscious" chapter of **Memories, Dreams, Reflection**, particularly the earlier parts, as the account of a journey whose outcome we don't already know. Jung felt profoundly isolated and alone as he found himself subjected to one frightening dream after another. Think of the dream of the corpses in the crematorium, of the dream of that long row of tombs dating back to the 12th century with the dead, one by one, coming back to life. Think of the dream of the bloody flood covering Germany, the arctic cold wave slowly freezing everything, the boulders that threaten to crush him. Think of Jung finding himself wading through sucking mud and then through icy water, the sun spurting blood, the chariot made of the bones of the dead. Think of how over and over again he feels himself being transported to the land of the dead.

What made it possible for him to sustain his commitment to this exploration was the creation of ritualized ways of working with these images and the emotions they evoked. He honored the power of those images with the meticulous renderings of the paintings in *The Red Book*. He wrote down the dreams in a deliberately chosen inflated style that he felt served to communicate their numinosity. He gave names to the figures that appeared in some of those dreams and then, wakingly, engaged them in conversation as a way of dreaming the dreams onwards. Sitting himself down on the beach in front of his lakeside home and playing in the sand, he experienced a recovery of the long-lost spontaneous playful creativity of his childhood. Discovering analogues between these dream images and games and the archaic myths and rituals he had discussed in his 1913 book The *Psychology of the Unconscious* (the book that in a later reworking became *Symbols of Transformation)* helped him realize that what he was undergoing was not just idiosyncratic or pathological or psychotic—but archetypal and meaningful. The ancient stories and rites also suggested that, though eventually there would be a re-emergence, it couldn't be hastened.

Slowly he began to hope that what he had undergone could be made meaningful for others by using what he had learned from his own experience to develop his own therapeutic rituals. This, he came to believe, might be the purpose of this almost six-year journey: that others might not have to undertake their forays so radically alone. So that, although their journeys would inevitably also be terrifying, dangerous, and sometimes seemingly endless, their fears about what they might encounter and their confusion about how to proceed, may be somewhat alleviated by being guided on the journey by someone who had made a similar one and could testify to the possibility that it might be more transformative than destructive—though, of course, no one can ever promise that. (I wonder though if anyone ever really does do this quite alone; there do always seem to be guides—or at least witnesses. Even Persephone had Hekate and Helios, Inanna had Ninshubar, Freud had Fliess, and Jung had Toni Wolff.).

When Jung began doing therapy again after the six year hiatus (though we know now from Deirdre Bair's biography that it wasn't quite as radical a hiatus as the somewhat romanticized account in **Memories, Dreams, Reflections** presents it), the therapeutic rituals he crafted were deliberately different in some ways from those he had learned from Freud. There are, of course, important commonalities: in both psychoanalysis and analytic psychology, during the therapy hour, we find ourselves in a world sharply set off from the world outside. We come at a set time each day or week; we come for fifty minutes or an hour. What happens in the consulting room belongs to an esoteric world; it is not to be spoken of outside, and makes little sense except to other initiates. We have entered a world where there are different rules, a different language, a different mode of temporality where past, present, and future melt into one another.

Admittedly, the rituals of Jungian therapy are in important and interesting ways different from those established by Freud. Nonetheless, they were created in relation to Freud's, so it behooves us to begin by looking at his. H.D.'s account of her analysis with Freud in her **Tribute to Freud** gives us a rich sense of its mythic and ritual aspect. She speaks of Freud as a midwife to the soul, as Asclepius the blameless physician, as an Orpheus who charms the very beasts of the unconscious and enlivens the dead sticks and stones of buried thoughts and memories . . . as an old Hermit who lives on the edge of the great forest of the unknown, as a trickster-thief nonchalantly unlocking vaults and caves and taking down the barriers that generations had carefully set up, as Faust, as a Prometheus stealing fire from heaven, as the curator in a museum of priceless antiquities.

It is fascinating to see how many of the typical features of initiation rituals are present in Freud's way of practicing analysis. For instance, nakedness: the "fundamental rule" of psychoanalysis is free association, the requirement that we say everything that enters our minds with no censorship, without the protection of cultural taboos or the expectation that what we say should make sense. Or, radical isolation: what happens in the consulting room is to be kept there, not brought outside, not discussed even with our closest others. Or, starvation: the analyst resolutely refuses to gratify the patient's hungers. Most importantly perhaps: silence and word magic.

Psychoanalysis is, after all, the "talking cure." Freud claims that speech itself, the right speech, heals; he invites his patients to free associate and thus to enter a new linguistic realm—an uncanny realm, unfamiliar and yet in some way deeply familiar. Every word calls for a reply and the analyst's silence is a reply, a reply that forces the patient toward free association. The analyst's silence keeps the patient's certitudes suspended, helps us discover that our being has never been more than an imaginary construct.

Without the silence there would not be the radical confrontation with ourselves that it forces upon us. But the silence is a silence within a world created by speech. Of course the analyst does speak, but first he listens—with evenly hovering attention, noticing not just what the patient says, but what he or she doesn't, noticing the silences, the gaps, the omissions, the repetitions. When he speaks it is to help us see how our speech conceals and not only reveals, how our longing for coherence, for narrative, for meaning, is evasive, how bent we are on hiding from ourselves.

The aim of therapy, so Freud believed, is to bring me into the world of words, and by way of words into the world of others. We become aware of self and (m)other as we enter language; thus language separates and is the medium of any later re-connection between self and other. Narcissism is death; communication, speech, is life.

The language of therapy is attuned to the erotic, the connective, aspect of language. It is talking with the other, Freud claims, that heals. Dialogue not introspection. This, of course, relates to Freud's emphasis on transference, on the ritual replaying of earlier relationships that occurs within the consulting room. Ritual is repetition; it is effective repetition, transformative repetition. Freud recognized that all love is transference love; we bring old patterns, old expectations, old fears to all our new relationships. We keep repeating the same old story but nothing happens. In analysis we are given the possibility of seeing, of experiencing, how the past lives on in the present and thus here repetition may become effective, transformative. Something might happen! These re-enactments, once recognized as re-enactments, make transformation possible (as mere intellectual understanding never will), because they give the patient an opportunity to experience the emotional charge still present in supposedly long outgrown childhood attachments.

Although Freud had already in his **Studies on Hysteria** noted the importance of the personal relationship between patient and physician, he had no inkling then that this could be understood as metaphorical incest—which of course is what "transference" is. Metaphor and transference are, after all, really the same word. The case of Dora led Freud to recognize that the failure of that analysis could be explained by his not making explicit Dora's projection of her father-longing onto Freud himself (and not only onto Herr K).

Psychoanalysis, he was beginning to see, somehow stirs up a re-enactment of the emotional patterns of the child's relation to its parents. He had earlier discovered the power of longings to shape our memories of the past; now he was discovering how those same longings operate to shape the present on the basis of that imagined version of the past. He saw how, unconsciously of course, we keep projecting the old patterns and longings onto new beloveds, and so don't really see them. There is no real *eros* connection, no real I-you engagement.

Henceforth working with the transference becomes the most important part of therapy. The transference feelings that he had at first looked upon as in the way of therapy become the way itself. Love, as he writes Jung at the time of the Spielrein crisis, is the medium of our work and sometimes we'll get burned. We cannot escape the risk of being scorched by the love with which we operate. The eros summoned up in the consulting room is dangerous; but to try to ignore would be to conjure up a spirit from underworld and then send it back without questioning it.

Though transference enters into all our relationships, what distinguishes what happens in treatment is simply that there it is provoked by the analytical situation and somehow intensified by the artificial context in which all taboos are lifted. Within analysis it is possible to bring into view the repressed elements of the relation to the parents: the erotic and the hostile aspects, not just the affectionate aspect of which the patient is already aware. The transference of this whole range of effects onto the therapist makes possible a transformation from literalism to an appreciation of the symbolic aspects of the incest complex, makes possible a realization that what was really wanted was transformation. not literal gratification.

In analysis, as Freud practiced, it is clearly the patient's love (not the therapist's) that is the source of healing; the analyst's compassion is expressed as dispassion. Freud invokes the incest taboo. In order to work the metamorphosis, the love evoked by therapy is to be admitted but not literally enacted. Its energy is needed to oppose all in the patient that resists cure; the longing for change, Freud believes, is in itself never strong enough. (It was in part this recognition that led Freud to his understanding of the role that death-wish plays in our lives.) Freud is deeply aware of how much psychic energy operates against therapy. He notes that if someone tries to take a neurotic's illness away from him, he defends it like a lioness with her young.

If the analyst were to respond directly to the patient's demand for his love, she would not have to get well. She would have been given what she thought she wanted but what is really an inadequate substitute for what she originally came to therapy for. Enactment would not free the patient from attachment to literalism: abstinence is intended to further metaphorical realization. Freud's central criticism of "wild" psychoanalysis was that gratifying their sexual desires deprives patients of the possibility of a real transformation of their way of being. Thus it is signally important that the analyst himself not take transference-love personally, literally, which is why he needs to have been through the process himself. (Freud is well aware how humanly difficult such abstinence can be, especially for a young therapist.)

Resolution of the transference can enable us to relate to the other as other, not just as a revenant of childhood attachment figures; the aim is to make it possible for us to love. The aim is not so much the elimination of the transference as its transformation, The goal is to make us more conscious, and appreciative of how the inevitable presence of our most powerful memories and expectations can lend depth, resonance, dimensionality to our present relationships. That is, we come to recognize that the new beloved is herself and my mother and my sister (and more mysteriously still, perhaps also my father.) The point is not to dissolve the imaginal facets, but to recognize—and celebrate—them as such.

Freud sought to free himself and his students and patients from transferring onto psychoanalysis our illusions of salvation. He voices his own skepticism concerning therapy from the very beginning. As almost everyone remembers, Freud once wrote that he saw the aim of therapy to be the transformation of neurotic misery into common unhappiness—a goal that I know sounds dismaying limited to some, but that I see as expressing the honesty and depth of Freud's understanding of our human being-here. Analysis, he believed, may help us become reconciled to Ananke, (necessity) and may teach us to take delight in our capacity for symbolization. It encourages us to acknowledge ambivalence, tolerate ambiguities, take delight in double meanings and in symbolic (that is, sublimated) satisfactions.

Jung, I believe, was more optimistic about what analysis has to offer. Speaking of himself vis-à-vis Freud, he once wrote: *I risked a greater shattering and achieved a greater wholeness.* I think he believed that his way of practicing analysis might help others toward a greater wholeness as well. One of the most obvious differences between the rituals of Jungian therapy from those of Freud is that in Jungian analysis the patient sits face to face with the therapist, rather than lying on a couch with the analyst out of sight. This yields a sense that analyst and patient are mutually engaged in the process. The analyst is present not as a blank screen but as a fellow human. When it's working, Jung says, something happens to both--and unless the analysts is open to himself being transformed, unless the analyst is fully present with all of his being, nothing important is likely to happen. It is easy to see that much is gained, but perhaps something is also lost: that radical, fearful confrontation with oneself that the free association rule imposes.

Instead of free association, there is conversation. In place of long-withheld interpretation, there is amplification, which may entail a tendency to move away from the details of the patient's images and conflicts to their mythological and archetypal analogues. Even transference is different or responded to differently. What is understood to be projected on the an-

alyst is less likely to be thought of as the literal mother or father of childhood but rather the archetype of Father or Mother, or perhaps of Savior
or Healer or Wise Old Man. Again much is gained by this shift away from
a focus on the personal, the pathological, the past—to the transpersonal,
the creative, the beckoning future. But again there may also be loss. So
much more attention is given to the discovery of inner riches than to
preparation for less wounded and wounding involvements with others.

Given these differences, it is nonetheless true that, for both Freud and
Jung, analysis is an initiation into underworld experience that may stir up
complex, ambivalent, ambiguous, contradictory fears and longings. We
enter a mysterious uncanny realm, an unknown and yet strangely familiar
world, the unconscious. This going forward seems in some sense to be a
return—a return to beginnings, to archaic understandings of the soul.

Jung's vision of the unconscious was in large measure shaped by a
dream in which he found himself continually descending from one floor
of a house to yet another more ancient one until at last he found himself
in an archaic underground cave surrounded by bones and pottery shards.
Freud begins **Interpretation of Dreams** with an epigraph from the Aeneid
in which Juno announces her resolve to turn to the underworld for help
the heavens have refused to grant her. Throughout the book, Hades, the
Greek underworld, serves as a metaphor for the unconscious. Hades is
not hell; it is a sacred realm ruled over by the goddess Persephone and her
consort, Hades. Many of the other gods and goddesses are also associated
with this realm and with underworld experience. The sacredness of the
underworld is something both Freud and Jung honored. Both knew that
what happened in analysis—when it happened—is not just the work of
analyst or analysand, but of what Buber called the "Between" or the spirit,
of *daimones* or gods.

At the very core of the rituals of depth psychology, of a psychology de-
voted to the soul, is the prayer: "May the Gods be present." Jung said that
the gods will be present, invited or not—but that inviting them in makes a
difference. Hillman has written about how important it is to know which
altar to approach, to know which god or goddess has brought our suffering upon us and thus which must be called upon for release. As the

Greeks knew, only the god who inflicted the wound can effect the healing.

The gods may make their presence evident in many different ways. They may appear in the person of the analyst (of course, it is important for both analyst and patient to know that the analyst isn't the god). In Greek mythology the gods often appear in human disguise, in the guise of a familiar other, a trusted mentor or even a suddenly glamorous husband. Or the god may appear as a figure in the patient's dream. Or as an energy in the room. Hermes, god of the lucky find, is clearly present in the room when-- after having arrived at an amazingly happy interpretation-- Freud tells H.D., "This deserves a cigar!"

Any of the gods or goddesses may appear. But those associated with *liminality*, with the crossing of the border between the upper and lower worlds, and those deities associated with the underworld itself, seem to be the ones whose presence we might most welcome as we find ourselves participating in the rituals of therapy. I have written more fully about who might be invited, in my **Journeys to the Underworld**.

May the gods be present. We need them all.

FACILITATING A RITUAL AND HEALING GROUP WITH PSYCHIATRIC CLIENTS

YARON PRUGININ

THIS ARTICLE DESCRIBES MY EXPERIENCE OF EXPLORING THE THERAPEUTIC powers of ritual-making in a long term residential facility. I started facilitating a Rituals
and Healing group in December 2005 at a psychiatric program in La Mesa, CA. My interest in this topic came from my ongoing involvement in different practices that applied rituals, such as martial and healing arts (Aikido and Shiatsu) and many Jewish and Native American rituals I have been exposed to over the years. These practices got me interested in taking a class on Rituals and Healing during my doctorate studies. The seminar focused on the therapeutic qualities of rituals in different cultures and through different theoretical prisms. Armed with that knowledge, but with no concrete idea of how to translate it into a therapeutic group setting, I embarked on a unique adventure.

In this paper I will share some of what I learned in that group. I will first outline the group setting and the structure we followed in each session. I will then describe some of the rituals that were created and performed in this group, followed by my understanding of their therapeutic value in the context of the individual's process of healing.

The Setting and Structure

I facilitated this group while working as a psychological assistant at Hanbleceya, a therapeutic program that provides intensive therapy (weekly or individual psychotherapy sessions and daily group sessions) and semi-independent living, supported by housing staff. The age of the clients in the program ranged from 19 to 65. All the clients in the program had severe psychiatric illnesses, such as schizophrenia, bipolar disorder, various addictions, mood disorders and personality disorders. The Ritual and Healing group met once a week, and was one of three groups that were offered simultaneously. Until that point, none of the ongoing groups addressed the clients' spiritual, religious and creative needs and abilities. This void, combined with my personal interests, led to the birth of the *Rituals and Healing* group.

The Group

Each 60-minute session was divided into 2 or 3 segments:

1) Opening and Grounding Rituals.

2) Ritual Development and

3) Ritual Performance (whenever a ritual was ready to be performed).

The Opening/Grounding Rituals (15-20 minutes): in this segment the group as a whole performed rituals that were meant to alert the members' consciousness, enhance their presence in the moment, and connect them with their bodies. We would begin with a Native American ritual of smudging, in which sage was burnt and passed around the circle. Then, still standing in a circle, we performed a movement meditation ritual that was based on Qi-gong exercises. Initially I introduced and facilitated these rituals. Later in the development of the group, group participants facilitated them on a voluntary basis.

Ritual Development (15-30 minutes): in this segment we used a Talking Stick that was passed from one group member to the next to indicate who was talking. During this time group members asked the group for support in creating their personal rituals. In the first sessions and whenever a new person joined, a handout with basic ideas regarding the use of rituals was reviewed. The amount of time that participants needed in order to create their rituals varied greatly, ranging from 2-3 weeks to several months. Group discussions allowed those participants who were better able to focus, and who had more resources and experience, to support those who were more easily overwhelmed by the task. Some participants needed more time to identify issues in their lives or events in their recent or distant past that they felt warranted a ritual. For these participants, the group provided guidance by asking questions and making suggestions.

An important tool to help participants develop their rituals was writing assignments that were prepared in advance and present to the group. In the initial stages, participants wrote about life-themes that they identified as meaningful to them. Later they would explore the meanings and relevance of the emerging themes to their current healing process. Finally, each participant would proceed to find ways to symbolize the theme and represent it in a concrete and structured way. For example, one participant identified that "letting go" was a life-long issue for him. Being a football fan, he created a ritual in which he threw a football around the circle, while naming things he would like to let go off (paranoia, bursts of anger, etc).

Since participation in the group was voluntary (participants could chose between this group and two other groups) I required active participation as a condition for group attendance. The rule was that anyone who did not prepare anything to present to the group for two consecutive weeks was asked to leave the group. Reentering the group was possible after discussing with me the reasons for not working in group and ways to overcome them.

Ritual Performance (15-30 minutes): the last segment of the group was dedicated to the performance of the rituals. Rituals varied greatly in complexity, length and topic. The simplest ritual, at least technically, was one performed by a psychotic 55 year-old man, who struggled for a long time to be able to stay in the room for the length of the session. After several weeks of discussion in the group he found the courage to bring a cassette with his favorite Beatles song and play it to the group. Other rituals involved more preparation and coordination. A 19-year-old participate used the group to motivate himself to write poems, which he then read to the group. These poetry readings evolved over time to include the group playing percussions to accompany the reading. Another ritual involved the burial of a guinea pig that had been the pet of one of the younger participants. She wrote a good-bye poem, made a drawing of her diseased pet, and found an appropriate burial site in her back yard. Following through on such specific and emotionally laden details of preparation was an important achievement for her: her main strategy of coping with strong unpleasant emotions had been self injury and substance abuse.

Some participants drew on their religious background to form rituals. For example, one participant who was in her thirties and who was brought up Catholic, created a Hail Mary ritual: she provided group members with rosaries, held a meditation with them, and read prayers at specific intervals. Another participant who was Jewish performed a Hanukkah ritual that included lighting the Menorah, telling the traditional story of the Maccabim and eating latkes that she had prepared in advance. On another occasion she performed a Yartzeit ceremony dedicated to the memory of her deceased parents. She used traditional candles and pictures of her parents to process her thoughts and feelings regarding her loss. For these participants, of great importance was the mere fact of successfully planning and executing an activity that involved their community members.

Charlie

One of the more elaborate rituals created in the group was created by a client who was recovering from a psychotic break and addiction to alcohol and marijuana. I will describe the development of his "sobriety sacrament" in some detail, in order to demonstrate the role of ritual performance in his particular healing journey. Charlie was a 25 year-old Caucasian male who had a psychotic break at age 18 and several more in his early twenties. He had an exceptional musical talent and had been practicing martial arts since childhood. During the peak of his illness, Charlie had tried to violently kill himself and was hospitalized twice in the course of three years due to persecution delusions and paranoia, symptoms that were exacerbated by his substance abuse.

When Charlie started the program, he presented as extremely anxious, particularly in social environments. He also had frequent bursts of anger.

Charlie chose to mark his first year of sobriety by performing a sobriety ritual. In preparation for the ritual, Charlie journaled about his experiences as an addict and later as an active AA member. Based on his own writings, he identified five stages in his journey. He then created a sacrament-like ceremony in which he read his journal entries for each one of those stages to the group, after which the group ate a food or a drink that he had chosen to represent that stage. Sour gummy bear candy represented his poignant experience when starting to use drugs; sweet gummy bears represented the "fun" stage of using drugs; white bread represented the ongoing stage of drug using, when the drug no longer had a strong effect on him; sparkling water represented his experience of being sober; finally, a selection of protein power bars, cranberry muffins and sourdough bread represented the choices he was making in the present between healthy and less healthy foods. During the ritual Charlie lay out all the foods on individual plates for each group participant. He then read from his journal, describing each stage of addiction. At the end of each reading all participants consumed the food, as in a sacrament.

On other occasions Charlie played his *tablas* (Indian drum) in rituals that marked his moving into independent living, a Christmas carol ritual, and a martial art breathing exercise ritual. Charlie also began to volunteer to lead the Qi Qong ritual at the beginning of group. Charlie's participation in the group demonstrated his creative talents and provided inspiration for other group members. His rituals and the role he took in supporting other participants to develop their rituals was part of a process in which Charlie became a leader within his community. I believe the ritual also had significance in reinforcing his determination to abstain from drinking alcohol or smoking marijuana.

About a year after he arrived at the program and participating in daily group sessions (*Ritual and Healing* being one of them) and weekly individual and family sessions, Charlie was enrolled in a community college and was taking music classes that will count toward a bachelor's degree in music.

Observations and Conclusion

Facilitating this group was a very powerful experience for me. I was repeatedly surprised by the creativity that the group participants uncovered -- and by the momentum of the group. The group started with four participants, with some sessions only two of them attending. By the end of my work at the program, the group had 10 regular participants. Another powerful component of the group was field trips to a local Native American sweat lodge ceremony, which had a surprisingly calming effect on those who attended them and provided a safe environment for social interaction in a non-structured setting.

Many authors have written about the therapeutic powers of rituals (Van den Hart, 1983; Butler, 1998). The most fascinating aspect of the Ritual and Healing group for me was finding practical and concrete ways to make the connections between each person's psychological and spiritual needs and rituals. In my training as a clinical psychologist I have received many teachings regarding the 'ritual' of psychotherapy as it has been practiced since its modern conception by Freud. This 'ritual' has been carefully looked at largely by therapists from the psychodynamic and psychoanalytic branches of psychotherapy, where routines and their disruptions are carefully looked at as they occur in the therapy office, in order to elicit meaning (McWilliams, 2004). The Ritual and Healing group expanded that horizon for me in the sense that it allowed me to utilize other sources of ritual. Accessing rich traditions such as Native American, Catholic and Jewish rituals helped us address psychiatric problems in the context of generations of human experience, not just the four walls of the clinic. I think that this connection was important in reducing the sense of isolation and shame that is often associated with therapy and that, in my opinion, often results in a more passive stance on the part of the clients. When creativity and spirituality entered the group room, I found myself and the participants accessing resources of imagination and creativity that may have not been accessible to us otherwise.

Additionally, research on the structure of the brain suggests that non-verbal activities can *greatly* help in accessing more instinctive parts of the brain and helping integrate them with the more verbal and voluntary parts (Koob & Le Moal, 2006). I believe that bringing mind-body practices and rituals into psychotherapy help achieve such integration.

References

Bickel, W. K. and Potenza, M. N. (2006) The forest and the trees: addiction as a complex self-organizing system, In: Miller, R. W. and Carroll, K. M (Eds). *Rethinking Substance Abuse,* New York, Guilford Press.

Butler, K. (1998). Beyond the Rational: Shamans, scientists and therapists join in a quest for meaning. *Family Therapy Network, 22 (9)* 24-37.

Koob, G.F. & Le Moal, M. (2006) The Neurobiology of Addiction. San Diego: Elsevier Academic Press

McWilliams, N. (2004). Psychoanalytic Psychotherapy: A Practitioner's Guide, New York, Guilford Press.

Van der Hart, O. (1983). *Rituals in Psychotherapy: Transition and Continuity.* New York, Irvington Publishers.

LACK OF FORMAL RITES OF PASSAGE FOR OUR HIGH-RISK YOUTH

DANA CARSON

As I LOOKED OVER THE LUSH EMERALD CANOPY FROM THE TEMPLE ATOP a pyramid in the middle of nowhere as if I had been here before, a familiar feeling passed through me. Although this was indeed my first visit to Tikal, the lush Mayan ruins of Guatemala, visions of an alternate time and another people flashed through my mind. No doubt influenced by a book I had read en route to the ruins: a virgin crawled up the steps to her last breath, in abeyance to the the Mayan kings' rule for community rituals of virgin sacrifice. In my reading, the text described a scenario barbaric and wasteful of life. However, as my feet carried me up the same stairs as hers had, and as I took in the view that melted into eternity as she had, a sliver of understanding of the community's beliefs in the power of such a sacrifice became less opaque. The grandiosity of the world and systems within which we are all just a small part was apparent. The immensity of this place radiated an intensity that can only be translated via experience . . . and ritual.

After taking in Tikal, I scanned my mental Rolodex of life experiences, searching for rituals or other peak experiences. A lack of rituals within my mainstream United States (U.S.) American culture was quickly apparent. Initially, I could only conjure up memories of church on Sundays, with weddings and funerals as the only outright rituals, sparse and ir-regular. Had I missed something? With clear relief to have avoided teen sacrifice, I still longed to know what life would be like in a culture closely bonded and bound by traditions and rituals. What might be missing in the lives of mainstream U.S. Americans because of our vanilla culture, with its lack of ritual?

As a U.S. American, I definitely enjoy my freedom to explore and self-discover, yet still, I cannot help but wonder if the current collective might be vying for a healthier direction if offered the wise guidance and structure of a ritually connected culture. What if our cultural road map had a few more explicit details? Would we be less lost, more worldcen-tric in our perspectives, enjoying the scenery more, and/or progressing further along the road? I decided to explore others' perspectives on these topics, particularly rites of passage, as a part of my graduate studies.

As I read further about rites of passage, a pleasant surprise emerged in that I identified a phase from my life that paralleled the process described by van Gennep (1960). Gennep (1960) initially described rites of pas-sage as consisting of three stages: a separation from one's previous societal role (i.e., no longer an adolescent); a liminal stage where one does not fully identify with a specific societal role (i.e. the developmental stage of emerging adulthood where one feels no longer adolescent, yet unsure about being an adult); and a reincorporation into one's newfound role (i.e. one is considered an adult).

This discovery granted me the realization that ritual had played a slightly more significant role in my development than revealed at first glance. Between the ages of 23 and 25, I lived in Nicaragua as a Peace Corps volunteer, training with a group of 19 other fearful, yet animated, U.S. Americans who were stepping into the unknown. I was aware of the embarkation being undertaken toward a life changing experience, but was unable to fathom the impact the people and life in a culture that was a drastic contrast to my own would impart upon me.

Initially considered *aspirantes*, or trainees, we spent close to three months living in small communities off the Pacific Coast Highway, each adopted by a Nicaraguan family who helped us learn to wash clothes on a concrete slab, directed us on how to bathe with a bucket, and kindly stoked the fire to warm and cook us food. It is an understatement that the lifestyle was extremely different than the comfortable one with which we were familiar. In my personal limbo, chickens and pigs walked through the house, and amoebas attacked my stomach, leaving me hospitalized my first week in country. I fumbled with communicating in a foreign language, as if a toddler. I had to dig deep within my heart and mind to understand why I had chosen this experience. I teetered between laughter and tears, as my daily work was reduced to the simple struggle of staying healthy, avoiding unpleasant latrine encounters, and practicing rolling rr's with my five year old Nicaraguan nephew (who had far superior skills). After completing the initial training in Spanish, agriculture, and Nicaraguan culture 101, we were initiated in a ceremony as *voluntarios de Cuerpo de Paz* (Peace Corps volunteers). This ceremony lacked personal investment from me at the time and carried the appearance of a formality, but in retrospect served as an invaluable initiation, for which I have delayed appreciation.

In retrospect, and in the context of Peace Corps as a rite of passage, my experience pushed me to expand on multiple developmental lines and propelled me to feel more pronounced as a human being. Upon return to U.S. soil, my feelings mingled between pride for the honor bestowed upon me by others, to estrangement due to my own sentiments of no longer knowing if I belonged in my own culture. Another stage of limbo ensued. Fears of feeling disconnected and potentially misunderstood by loved ones held me captive as I tried to understand how to reincorporate into my culture and community. My societal role felt unclear.

Eventually, a job working primarily with Latinos with mental illness materialized, and I slowly, but successfully, reintegrated into U.S. culture. While no one said to me, "You're an adult now" upon my return, I felt greater awareness and an increased responsibility to serve others. A shift that happens between adolescence and adulthood is a movement from egocentric to being increasingly selfless. I recognized that my "pre-Nicaragua-experience, somewhat-service-oriented personality" had evolved. Having been on the outside and seeing the world through a new lens left me wondering what U.S. Americans were seeking in life, particularly during maturation, as some friends and acquaintances appeared stagnant, still engaging in college-like antics. I also wondered about how/why our country continues to deteriorate in regards to social and global problems, even though affluence abounds.

Campbell (1988) and Shepard (1982) both expounded upon the theory that lack of ritual in U.S. mainstream culture has led many adolescents to seek their own rites of passage. These gentlemen conjectured that many of the high-risk behaviors in which we see youth engage, often the root of societal dismay, are attempts at seeking a rite of passage. Looking at my own experiences, particularly while in Nicaragua, I engaged in both destructive and constructive high-risk behaviors, including late nights at the disco, hitchhiking alone, and/or riding on top of old school buses as a preferred method of transport to traverse the country. In retrospect, these high-risk behaviors were ways to release developmental stress, connect with others, and push myself to feel empowered. In consideration of this theory (that adolescents act out from a lack of ritual), I wanted to understand the developmental process from adolescence to adulthood. My studies led me to seek out individuals without formal rites of passage, to understand whether self-initiated or informal rites of passage prevailed.

The Maturational Process, Ambivalence Around Adulthood, and the Adolescent Societal State within the United States

One could easily spend lifetimes pondering the developmental role of ritual, or lack thereof. I spent several years reading related materials and ultimately conducted my own research on the topic. In focusing on the maturation process, specifically the transition from adolescence to adulthood, there are distinct shifts in today's society as compared with a few generations past. Adolescence itself has been dubbed a period of self-exploration and a quest for one's identity, as defined by Erik Erikson (1968). While past literature suggested the next developmental phase to be adulthood, a new stage of *emerging adulthood* has been proposed (and largely accepted) as an interim stage preceding adulthood in industrialized nations (Arnett, 1994, 2000, 2003; Shulman, Feldman, Blatt, Cohen, & Mahler, 2005). For emerging adults, the process of identity development continues and includes an extensive period of time before marrying, engaging in the work force, and/or having children. Emerging adulthood is thought to begin around age 18 and continue through the twenties.

My research explored the developmental trajectory as it pertained to ten individuals from Generation X, who were between the ages of 30 and 34, the most recent generation to have passed through the chronological stage of emerging adulthood. None of these individuals had a formal rite of passage to signify a transition to adulthood, such as a bar mitzvah or quinciñera. Recognition of a sense of adulthood was present, as identifying as an adult was an inclusion criteria, but an underlying ambivalence to take on the "adult" label was also evident.

Arrival to adulthood is a complex process. Most participants felt they evolved to adulthood (largely defined by responsibility specific to one's actions, fiscal management, and emotional maturity) over time, rather than becoming an adult at a specific age. The multi-layered sense of adulthood articulated the complexity of society and development as a contributor to the ambivalence to claiming adulthood. Recognition by others that one had reached the role of "adult" typically happened before these GenXer participants themselves felt like adults. Being treated respectfully when making purchases in a store or by a stranger, or encouragement of increased self-reliance by parents, were mentioned as sources of when participants felt seen as adults.

In addition, connotations about becoming an adult were a mixed bag. Freedom to do what one wanted, including eating ice cream before dinner, made adulthood appealing. But participants also perceived adulthood as "boring", being about paying bills in a doldrum routine, as if adults became mindless robots in the rat race of life.

You should be married with children by now. This societal expectation was perceived generally by participants who were not married with children, and appeared necessary for them to completely and truly be accepted as an "adult." This expectation especially resulted in feelings of disappointment, lack of achievement, and ambivalence.

Marriage and parenthood involve obvious role changes that continue to be easily observed within U.S. society and are marked by enduring rituals, such as weddings and baptisms. Without marriage and children, without ritual markers for the community and culture to recognize adulthood, these participants experienced ambivalence about notions of adulthood

Means to a Brighter Future

The U.S. society itself has been described as adolescent (Campbell, 1988; Plotkin, 2008). This societal "center of gravity" leaves children and future generations without the important mentorship and modeling that might help society to advance. The participants in my study mentioned cultural figures that modeled early adolescence (Common classroom characters such as Twain's Huckleberry Finn and Salinger's Holden Caulfield, struggling to integrate into society). They found them more influential in their perceptions of becoming an adult than stories that evoke completion of the *monomyth* of the hero's journey (Campbell, 1949). The mythological pattern parallels the steps taken in a formal rite of passage: a young person heeds the *call to adventure*, faces challenges that serve as initiations, receive guidance and help from unsuspected sorts, and then returnin to share the wisdom. One cannot help but wonder, if U.S. cultural mythological figures like Caulfield and Huck hold ambivalence regarding adulthood, whether they mirror a society's arrested development.

In consideration of the implications of an adolescent society and our lack of (or dispensable) formal rites of passage, a concern is unavoidable. While the U.S. has done well in some facets in the global community, social issues beg for attention, particularly those involving youth. Apart from substance use and risky sexual behavior, criminal activity and violence are high-risk behaviors with an alarming prevalence in the U.S. American adolescent population.

Feeling hopeless, helpless, and deflated yet? Well, the concern cooked up in considering these societal ills can be calmed to some degree by a review of interventions employing rites of passage framework to deter such adolescent issues. A major contributor to the literature and prominent practitioner in the use of rites of passage with adolescents is Blumenk-rantz (1992, 1996). He operates a Connecticut center called the "Rites of Passage Experience (ROPE)", which focuses on creating rites of passage within the community. The program generally has a duration of three phases throughout six years. Parent/Guardian involvement is essential and included in the formation of the rituals and mentorship for the youth. ROPE has proven to prevent substance abuse and delinquency, increase family involvement, and promote a sense of community and attachment to school.

Blumenkrantz's (1992) programs have successfully created the neces-sary phases of rites of passage (specifically separation, mentorship, tran-sition, and a welcoming from the community) to support adolescents' movement toward adulthood; these interventions are yielding positive results. While ritual and myth in U.S. culture seem to be losing potency vs the scream of daily headlines, these programs suggest some resolution. They deliver rejuvenation of rites of passage ceremonies and ritual, in-cluding the elements of community and mentorship. Small collectives, such as those being developed by the ROPE program, are pushing to re-thread ritual and myth into the tapestry of U.S. American society. An-cient ways can lead to a path of reconnection with our youth and can effectively allow a rebirth of wisdom.

Participants in my study, particularly males, felt that more mentor-ship would have been beneficial in their development. All these men had fathers present (who they considered mentors), but they desired further guidance. This speaks to a universal and essential need for community, from which mentorship for adolescents can blossom. Those of us who are adults must consider means that we can mentor youth, with the men-torship package incorporating community, whether formal or informal. A key finding in my study-- that others seeing them as an adult occurred before participants' themselves felt like an adult-- suggest that we must impart expectations of responsibility upon our youth in order for them to flourish and advance.

More generally, we can all choose from a plethora of opportunities to support agencies that are striving to improve society and lift us out of our adolescent haze. We as a whole can put energy toward the further maturation of our society so that mentors and community are able to pull us forward to initiate an increasingly sustainable world, for our youth and for ourselves.

CREATIVITY AS A RITUAL OF CHANGE IN HIGH RISK YOUTH

WES CHESTER

PREFACE

FOR MANY YEARS NOW, I HAVE BEEN TEACHING IN MY FIELD OF EXPRESSIVE Arts Therapy, at both the graduate and post-graduate level. I had worked with children as young as five in therapeutic inpatient settings, and also with teens and adolescents in psych hospitals. In the fall of 2008, I accepted an opportunity to teach a less familiar population: at-risk adolescents. It was an opportunity to work in my own studio space, for a program I believe in.

The adolescent population comes with its own unique challenges. Those challenges are compounded when the students are labeled as troublemakers or bad kids.

The students come to my studio from the ALBA (Alternative Learning for Behavior and Attitude) School, a school of last resort for those who have been removed from the normal classroom for violation of the district's Zero-Tolerance Policy towards weapons, violence or controlled substances. Their offences can range from carrying a pocketknife to dealing drugs. The staff of ALBA are dedicated, patient and vigilant. They work with a system of behavioral rewards, and most students are able,

with time, to return to a regular classroom. Students demonstrating adequate behavior Monday to Thursday may attend alternative classes on
Fridays.

And Fridays is where the Liberty School and the Expressive Arts Institute comes in. The stated mission of the Liberty School is to provide an
educational experience which is "...less constrained than the traditional approaches to public education ... " and to "... foster creativity." It was daunt-
ing to imagine how I could help students who had been selected out of
their normal classrooms by their own behavior. In my one hour per week,
I would need to offer something engaging, challenging and seductive to
these students. As I considered the needs of the population, an idea began
to emerge. What these kids needed was a way to reintegrate into a culture
which has clearly labeled them Other. What they needed was a ritual to
heal the rift between them and the culture, the education system, and each
other. It seems like a ridiculously tall order, that one ritual could undo a
lifetime of conflict with the community and each other, and a six-year history of struggle in school. But ritual needs uncertainty and risk.

THE POPULATION

The Zero Tolerance club is a largely male affair, perhaps because of
the unsuitability of the structure of education for young men. It isn't hard
to imagine how the boys I teach get into trouble. They are frenetic and
loud, boisterous, wrestling, shoulder-punching, and name-calling. They
disdain anything quiet and still. Even when they contemplate, it is always
as a precursor to action. They are thirteenish, on the cusp of adolescence,
some already taller than me, others not to my shoulder. They are Latino and Black, Asian, Pacific Islander, Native American, White, Indian,
and Arabic. The more developed boys practice an icy cool reserve, barely
dragging their bodies from place to place, sitting or lounging at every
opportunity. The younger ones are fighting gravity, bouncing on the balls
of their feet, rocking in their chairs, leaping and running at the slightest
provocation. And they make an art of provoking each other. They are

living out a tradition at least 20,000 years old; the young warrior testing his strength, establishing a pecking order, railing against restraint, and trying his best to uproot tradition.

In a culture which places a high value on peace and stability (at least domestically), these young warriors are a dangerous species. In an educational culture which values compliance, their behaviors signal a dangerous non-conformity. These are boys moving quickly towards the watershed beyond "trouble", when Juvenile Hall will become jail. Impulse control problems will give way to violence or addiction. The lack of significant connection to community will be replaced by gangs and turf wars.

An Objective

As a baseline, ritual must serve a visible purpose, else it is an empty choreography. That purpose may be wholly imaginal or it may be entirely concrete, but it must be real. In tribal culture, the transition to manhood is one marked by ritual rites of passage and initiations, which transform not only the individual, but the role in culture. Boys do not become men, or girls women, based upon age. They must learn to use the tools of the tribe, and do the work of the tribe. They must face trials which are dangerous, to learn the secrets of the tribe. They must learn the code of behavior for membership. In a village, this is not difficult. There, they are surrounded by elders and relatives.

The boys in my village have no common culture. Allegiance falls along lines of race, school, neighborhood, favorite team or band, favorite brand of shoe. Their only common bond is a failure to comply with the system set up for their schooling. So our ritual must be one in which everyone is equally alien, equally equal. We must enter the liminal space of ritual transformation together.

I have fourteen boys for thirteen hours in fifteen weeks. There is precious little time. And I have chosen a task which I am not sure can be achieved: To build an orchestra, a musical tribe.

The community relationship will be built in two ways. First through the guild of the maker, the crafts person, the apprentice. The boys will design the musical instruments, will make them with real tools in real time. Second they will learn to play their instruments, not in the childhood tradition of learning blithe, folksy melodies. They must learn to bring new music, never before heard, into being.

Making any object, be it an artwork or a blanket, teaches self-reliance. But making a tool to do other work with, such as an instrument to make music with, is a higher order of task. If a student has been expelled for secretly carrying a knife to school, what better thing to do than to require them to use a knife, safely, responsibly and constructively. In similar fashion, making improvisational music is communication on the highest order. For boys who have trouble communicating, improv teaches attention, with listening a necessity. And improv also engenders cooperation, and acknowledgment of the shared aesthetic experience.

This plan offers a clear risk of failure, ranging from vague dissatisfaction all the way to catastrophic injury. And it must be so. In the tradition of rites of passage, any trial must offer at least the opportunity, if not the certainty, of failure. And it must also provide space to seek support and guidance from the elders. The structure of the ritual must offer a place where initiates may also take responsibility for their own actions and safety. Real skills must be taught, and the making must be serious. It is of great importance that the initiates understand the difference between assuming a role, and acting. They will be reminded again and again that "Musicians play, but they don't pretend." The experience of making an instrument and then performing an original composition on that instrument must be one of the rarer experiences of our culture. When we acknowledge the power of authorship in our own aesthetic life, then our imagination is no longer bounded by the mass-produced image. Assuming responsibility for our diet of images is a beginning to live as a response-able person, contributing our cultural conversation.

ELEMENTS OF RITUAL

Rituals are not magic. They can vary from a birthday celebration to combat. But they all come with a short list of necessary ingredients.

There must be a clear transition into the ritual space from everyday life.

The experience must be non-ordinary, and must be identified as such by the facilitator. Actions within the ritual space take on a greater weight, by virtue of their metaphoric content. The reasons for doing things in the ritual space must not be purely mechanical. (Birthday candles are not lit for light, but specifically to be snuffed.)

The ritual must come with clear, hierarchical guidance, and boundary setting. The neophyte cannot be left unguided in the ritual space. Only as experience is gathered, can the participant begin to take on self-directed roles in the ritual.

The ritual must come with a clear way to return to ordinary experience.

Finally, for rites of passage, there must be something more. There must be a challenge to be overcome. And there must be an element of transformation of the person and his role.

Liminality and the Transition to Non-Ordinary Experience

The ritual space is actually my studio. As they arrived, two groups of potential students were required to remove their shoes, to come to a circle, and come to silence. As simple as it sounds, this transition to non-ordinary did focus the boy's attention for the initial message. This evocation of the work begins by identifying the non-ordinariness of the experience, as paraphrased here:

You have come to this place, apart from your family and your school, to undertake a task. At the end of our time, the task will be done, and you will be someone new, different than you are now. The task is not easy. We will learn the secrets for designing and making real instruments with real tools to play real music. We will end with a performance on those instruments, in front of your peers and parents. To become an adult, you must learn to use the tools of the tribe, and do the work of the tribe, and you must learn the songs of the tribe. When you are done, you will be a member of the tribe of makers, and the tribe of musicians. The task is dangerous. The tools we will use are real and powerful, and capable of producing life-threatening injuries. What will keep you safe is to obey your tribal elders without question. When you are asked to stop what you are doing, stop.

Through this statement, the boys were given information that they were entering a non-ordinary task, one which promised some challenge, change and transformation.

When I got my first look at the students who would follow the ritual through the remainder of the program, I began a new routine. The students arrived in the hallway with the doors closed and locked. Their knocking would summon me to the door only after some rattling of the handle, and pressing of the face to the frosted glass panel. At this point, I would exit the studio into the hall, and call them to silence with the ringing of the *ting-sha*, the small Tibetan meditation bells. Then I addressed them with the objectives for the day, reminding them of the rules of the studio, before we entered. The content of the hallway speech varied with each meeting, but contained these elements.

--An assessment of the previous weeks' successes and challenges.

--A reminder of the authority of the tribal elders (myself and the other teachers) in all matters.

--An assignation of responsibility to the initiates (students) for the outcome of the day.

--An invocation to do good work, and to keep their peers safe.

--Crossing the threshold (the literal *lim* of liminality), for the work of the day to begin.

The Necessity of Fear

The function of challenge in a rite of passage is to allow the sense of mastery, critical to the assumption of a new role in the community. The mastery most often addressed in a rite of passage is the mastery of one's own fear. As such, rites are prone to unpredictable and novel encounters, many of which depend upon theatrics. My version of this was to introduce new and "dangerous" tools at each meeting.

To begin the building phase of our class, I greeted them with the most imposing tool in the arsenal. I managed to capture the absolute wide-eyed attention of the planet's most jaded audience. Fourteen adolescent boys granted the absolute silence due a to bearded stranger revving a live power tool. Silence deepens as the blade spins down after the gravely roar of the motor. Spoken Clint Eastwood style: "This is a 7 ¼ inch circular saw, with a 15 amp motor that spins a tungsten-carbide tipped high-speed steel blade nearly a hundred times a second. It could take your finger off before you know you're cut." For the boys, few of whom had ever encountered a power tool, it was a jaw dropping moment. "You will need all your fingers to finish your work." Nervous laughter. But also attraction.

By the class end, we had the necks for our instruments cut, and a pile of useless small blocks, produced because everyone needed to use the circular saw at least once.

I became the coach guaranteeing safety and success. Boys came with clinched jaws, eyes squinting behind safety glasses as they pulled the trigger. Slouching coolness is impossible to maintain with a running saw in your hand. Seeing and hearing the saw rip through the board, while sawdust sprays over your shoes, and smelling the slightly spicy aroma of kiln dried poplar are decidedly non-virtual experiences. Faces became a little more serious.

When a small, slight boy stepped up to the table, looks were passed around. Someone stepped forward to offer advice. "I got it man," he replied casually. As with all the other boys, I told him only to "make the pencil line disappear." Unlike everyone else so far, Angel did. His cut was quick, but not rushed, dead straight, and done without swagger. The saw stopped, and I held the stick of poplar out for his group to see. "Now, that will do." An almost imperceptible smile from Angel, who nodded and stepped aside for the next boy. But Angel had just turned the pecking order upside down, and over the coming weeks he would become one of the leaders in building the instruments.

Over the weeks, the boys gained mastery over jigsaws and high-speed drills, hole-saws and razor knives, chisels, hacksaws and soldering irons, and a dozen other tools. Over the weeks, only one scratch, too small for a Band-Aid. Certainly mistakes were made. Holes drilled in the wrong place. Parts epoxied on backwards, screws stripped, wood split. We problem solved together. I began to let the boys decide what needed to be done next to meet their design requirements. They were becoming part of the ritual, suggesting the clean-up time, and insisting on tools getting back into their proper place (At the end of the course, no tool had disappeared -- not because of my vigilance, but because they watched each other).

VALIDATION OF THE WORK AND THE RETURN TO ORDINARY EXPERIENCE

At the end of each class, I used the same simple structure. First a series of questions, to bring the ritual space to a close. "Who did something they never did before today? Who used a tool they never used before today?" Hands were raised, and a few shared experiences. Next the lore befitting whatever tools were used. "The saw is the tool we use to divide things, to make the parts we need to create the whole. The drill is the tool our tribe uses to make holes, the empty space that allows us to make connections, from inside to outside, or between parts. These are the tools of our tribe." The boys would look at the work accomplished in the day, for which I would congratulate them. In this way, I reinforced the idea of tools as a connection to the tribe.

Finally, to part company, always the same benediction. "Makers, we have done a lot, but there is a lot to be done. I will need you all to come back next week. And how do you get to come back?"

"Good behavior."

"Don't let me down. Go out and have a good weekend, and a good week."

Of course, they did "let me down" from time to time. In some classes there were only six or eight. But for the most part, the boys worked hard to participate. And along the way there were small victories. On one particular day, the institute hallways were full of art for our annual show. As I gathered the boys in the hall, I pointed out some intricately decorated metal footlockers. "Those pieces were done by a homeless kid, about your age."

A redheaded boy with pale skin mumbled under his breath, "Must've had too much time on his hands." Not getting a sufficient reaction from his peers, he said it again.

"I heard you the first time," I replied quietly. Speaking quietly is one of the keys to communication with adolescent boys. And silence can be even more powerful.

Finishing the weekly check-in, I made sure to put the young critic into a leadership role for the day. Together, we worked out how to use a nail and a strip of cardboard to mark out a perfect circle on the wood for the face of a harp. At the close of the hour, when I gave my closing spiel, the redheaded boy hung back, approaching me shyly. "Mr. Chester. I can't come back next week. My dad is taking me camping." I nodded. "But can I come back the week after that?"

"I require it." And he did come back.

Closing Ceremonies

The instruments were done by week ten. Our orchestra consisted of six three-string cigar box guitars, a 12-string box slide guitar, and a strange, circular harp, designed with a water-bottle resonator. At this point, I announced that the period of making was done, and that the ceremony as musicians was close by. This transition was planned for Parents Day, where I would give a few minutes to explain our process, announce them as instrument makers and musicians, the boys would perform a song.

But as often happens in untried structures, wrinkles emerged. The eleventh week, the first week of rehearsal, three girls showed up. Not only were the boys distracted by their presence, but when the girls were asked to participate in the music making, they demurred and mugged, giggling at each other and the boys, whispering back and forth. They effectively "stonewalled" the rehearsal. Finally I divided the class into groups, with a sitting half including the girls out as audience. This helped a little, and with time running down, we finally performed a piece which took hold. There was a call and response between instruments, and the piece traveled, as a soundscape. When the boys and girls left, I was pacing the floor for a while, trying to solve the challenge of restoring some connection to the ritual. It would take me a week, and some luck, to work this out.

Fridays are at a premium in my studio, because my graduate students usually meet there. On the Wednesday before my last class, the grad students were in rebellion, not wanting to be displaced again by meeting at a local restaurant for breakfast lecture. Finally it hit me. The women, studying the arts as social and political responsibility, needed a place to be. I needed more tribal elders, and ceremonies need witnesses. A rite of passage does not welcome you into a theoretical community. It can't take place in an imaginary village.

So, on the final morning, I brought the six boys and one girl (the rest absent due to behavior issues) in and sat them down on cushions, before a row of empty chairs. "This morning, we will have visiting elders. They will examine and play your instruments." The grad students, eight women, filed in, taking their place in the chairs, where they were handed instruments. The kids were quiet, watching carefully as the women inspected their work. Instruments were touched, plucked, struck, strummed, turned over in their hands. Smiles began to appear, with oohs and wows and words of approval. The makers sat taller. After a couple of minutes, I called the elders to attention as musicians, giving them a simple structure for getting in and out. "We will begin in silence."

The rhythm arose slowly, building into a rich harmonic tapestry. The cigar box guitars, tuned as dulcimers, and the drone of the box slide, hummed over a pulsing rhythm. And the musicians were quickly entrained with the rhythm, allowing themselves to be led. The women, having never touched the instruments before, created a beautiful piece, allowing the makers for the first time to hear the potential of the instruments they had made. There was spontaneous and real applause at the ending. The instruments were pronounced good.

"And now, we switch places." The boys and girl take the stage. "Same structure," I say, "beginning in silence. Entering one at a time. Letting each one find his or her place, before the next comes in." The piece is loose at first, and descends, after a couple of minutes, finally coming to a halt. I ask the value neutral question, "In this piece, what is working and what isn't?" Many observations are made, but the one which strikes me comes from the audience. "Brittany didn't play at all. I wonder why?" Sitting center stage, she had not even attempted to hold her instrument up. Brittany demurred, but the women were insistent. "Come on, you are the representative for the women here, you can't let us down."

When we began again, the piece found coherence immediately. And Brittany joined in, began to smile, and have fun. She needed the support of these wise elders. The piece worked brilliantly, becoming a soundtrack, slowly building tempo, until it reached a driving pace, sounding like a raga. Finally, it reached a crescendo, and then slowed, fading instrument by instrument into silence. It was a piece which had every element of complex composition. Melodic and rhythmic movement, changes in dynamic, timbre and tempo, all played with serious engagement. The applause caught the musicians by surprise. They seemed suddenly a bit embarrassed, but very pleased to be greeted with appreciative attention. My expert witnesses gave feedback in great detail, pointing out the role each musician had played, and what they liked with specificity. My young makers soaked it up.

"And now, it is time for the ceremony. Elders form two lines here, facing one another. Musicians stand. You have joined the tribe of makers and musicians. When something needs building, you will stand ready to help. And when someone calls for musicians, you will step forward. Musicians, walk between us. Elders, welcome our new members."

The young musicians are beaming and blushing, walking forward, greeted by applause and cheers, pats on the back, words of encouragement. And after they have passed through, the applause continues, until they circle once again through the line as in a blessing. A moment of sweetness passes between us, all open, smiling, blushing. For this moment, they are of us, and we also belong to them. They are the young pride of our tribe. We take our parting gently, with praise and encouragement, and their promises not to meet again in Alternative Learning school. I send them forth with something akin to hope.

The next day is parents' day. The studio is spotless, the instruments arranged on a gold cloth, the tools used to make them laid out in neat ranks. No parents arrive. My new tribe is, it seems, adrift. In the hall I greet our director Susan, looking worried. She has been up all night. A student in our sister program has just gone down for armed robbery at age 16, tried as an adult, and is going away for 15 years without parole. The rites of his new tribe will include the irretrievable loss of youth. She leaves me to pack away my tools. I cannot stand to store the instruments. They are rough and lively, and beautiful. I wanted them to be seen and handled awhile before they are sent to storage. I pick up a cigar box guitar, painted like a Mexican flag, and play for a long time, wondering what will become of these young makers. Is there any protective magic in being heard, being held in belonging by a community of elders, even for a brief hour? What, if anything, can be saved through this simple ritual of bringing attentions. What hope can be held by this fragile talisman, this instrument of wood and skinny wires, softly singing in my hands?

CONTRIBUTORS

ALKIN, MELIS

Dr. Alkin received her doctorate degree in Clinical Psychology from CSPP in 2004 and was certified by the American Board of Professional Psychology as a Diplomate in Clinical Psychology in 2007. Between 2004 and fall of 2008 she lived and worked in Istanbul, Turkey where she had a private practice, taught at Bosphorous and Dogus Universities, and under Helsinki Citizen's Assembly's Refugee Legal Assistance Program, founded and directed mental health services program for asylum seekers and refugees living in Istanbul, Turkey. She currently has a private practice in the North Vancouver, B.C providing psychotherapy to adolescents and adults Dr Alkin has also been serving as an Adjunct Faculty and Research Ethics Board member at Adler School of Professional Psychology, Vancouver since January 2010.

BEACH, ELVA MAXINE

Elva Maxine Beach was born to a family of preachers, teachers, and storytellers. The psyche-sexual dramas that have become Beach's oeuvre are the subject of her first book length publication, Neurotica. This short story cycle is a provocative collection of explicit stories chronicling the narrator's intimate journey from sensual awakening to spiritual transcendence. "I wanted to capture the reality of my own spiritual travels through a fictionalized accounting of the sexcapades I have both lived and imagined." Neurotica was published by New Belleville Press in June 2008 (newbellevillepress.com). Beach is currently Associate Professor of English at St. Louis Community College at Meramec.

BUSBY, J. REBECCA

Dr. Busby has an incisive wit that can reveal the truth and expose the humor in our human condition. A positive attitude assists us in facing and accepting our limitations. Her own story is one of courage, strength, and wisdom. She has lived with Rheumatoid Arthritis and Sjogren's Syndrome for 30 years. She maintains a positive attitude in her life despite decades of chronic illness. Her specialties include: Emotional Distress Issues, Coping Strategies, Health and Wellness, Palliative Care, Spirituality, and Gratitude. Along with her academic accomplishments, she possesses an insightful intuition in working with her clients. Dr. Busby is gifted in her ability to explain her insights to her clients in a non-threatening, and engaging discourse.

Cappadonna, Dominie

Building upon 30 years post-doctoral work in the field of Ecopsychology, Transpersonal Psychology and Education, I am delighted to bear witness with transformations of all kinds, through teaching and offering a private practice as a psychotherapist, and ecopsychologist. As a wilderness therapy, ecopilgrimage and expeditions guide, I have led journeys in wild places by land and sea for 27 years. I am grateful to translate ecopsychological principles and practices in trans-cultural social action training with in Brazil, China, and Cambodia. I work as a facilitator for Joanna Macy's "Work that Reconnects" and am trained in Ken Wilber's Integral Sustainability practices. I am committed to engaged spirituality, in all its' forms.

Carroll, Michael

Michael Carroll is a licensed psychologist. He lives in Encinitas, California with his beautiful wife Julie and two brilliant daughters, Chloe and Lily

Carson, Dana

Culture and people are two creatures with which I have always been fascinated. My curiosity has taken me around the globe from parts of Europe to Latin America, from South East Asia and India to Russia. These experiences have led me to try to gain a better understanding of my cultural background that used to seem so [3]normal[2] until I was able to step outside of it. My other interests involve the outdoors, running, biking, swimming, creating and enjoying art, getting my hands in the dirt, and passing time with friends and family. I completed the Clinical Psychology PsyD program at Alliant International University in the fall of 2009, and pursue work with children and families, as well as providing care to underserved populations.

Chester, Wes

Wes Chester, MA, CAGS, Expressive Arts Therapist, is an outdoorsman, artist, musician, instrument maker and poet, who has been facilitating the arts for healing and change since 1996. His master's thesis introduced Expressive Arts to the concept of Eco-Aesthetics, an arts and philosophy based understanding of healing through the sensual encounter with nature. In addition to teaching, and private practice, he manages the Bayview Clubhouse a milieu therapy program for persons with severe mental illness. Wes is the co-director of the Expressive Arts Institute, in San Diego, CA a graduate school focused upon teaching through the embodied experience, and peer supported learning in an environment of scholarly inquiry. www.arts4change.com

Davis, John

John Davis, Ph.D, teaches the Diamond Approach through the Ridhwan School and leads wilderness retreats and trains wilderness rites of passage guides as a staff member of the School of Lost Borders. A former department chair and director of programs in Transpersonal Psychology and Ecopsychology at Naropa University, he is currently an adjunct professor there. John is the author of The Diamond Approach: An Introduction to the Teachings of A.H. Almaas (Shambhala). He has a special interest in exploring the interweaving of nature, psyche, and spirit, first-hand in wilderness and his garden as well as conceptually.

Dombrowe, Christian

I am a licensed Clinical Psychologist trained at the prestigious Ruprecht-Karls-University of Heidelberg. My special focus during my

M.A. was Clinical Psychology and Psychosomatics. Upon completion of
the PhD-program in East-West-Psychology I have been awarded a Ph.D.
by the California Institute for Integral Studies in San Francisco. My training at CIIS has added an integrative, holistic understanding to my clinical
practice. My therapeutic approach has been influenced by Intercultural
and Contemplative Psychotherapy. I am aware of the crucial importance
of intercultural competence and communication when working with people from diverse cultural backgrounds. I completed my Postgraduate Psychodynamic Psychotherapy training at the Berlin Academy of Psychothe.

Downing, Christine

Christine Downing, currently a Professor of Mythological Studies at
Pacifica Graduate Institute in Santa Barbara, taught for almost twenty
years in the Department of Religious Studies at San Diego State University and Core Faculty at the San Diego campus of the California School
of Professional Psychology. From 1963 to 1974 she served as a faculty member of the Religion Department at Douglass College of Rutgers
University She has also taught at the Jung Institut in Zurich and lectures
frequently to Jungian groups both here and abroad and at American and
European universities. . Her undergraduate degree in literature is from
Swarthmore College; her Ph.D., in religion and culture is from Drew University Her books include The Goddess; Journey Through Menopause,
Psyche's Sisters, Myths and Mysteries of Same-Sex Love, Mirrors of the
Self, Women's Mysteries, Gods In Our Midst, The Long Journey Home,
The Luxury of Afterwards, d Preludes: Essays on the Ludic Imagination,
and Gleanings.

Eulert, Don

Don Eulert, Ph.D., studied at the C.G. Jung Institute Zurich as a poet,
not as psychologist. His interest in cultural mythology and participation
in rituals has taken him from Romania to Kenya, from the Navajo Nation
to Thailand. For 40 years he has emplaced in the back country of San
Diego County on land that was a stop point for the migratory Ipay tribe.

FLEURIDAS, COLLETTE

Colette Fleuridas, Ph.D., currently a professor in the Graduate Counseling Program at Saint Mary's College of California, has been the department chair for ten years (at SMC and at CSU Chico, where she taught in the Department of Psychology for five years), and has been in clinical practice in a variety of settings for ten years. Her research web page is www.spiritresearch.org, where she gathers data about peoples' spiritual and religious beliefs, practices, values and experiences. In addition to spending time with family and friends, she enjoys traveling, landscaping, yoga, hiking, backpacking, and cross-country skate skiing.

HABIB, TOM

Thomas A. Habib, Ph.D. is a clinical psychologist practicing at Thomas A. Habib, Ph.D. & Associates in San Juan Capistrano, California. For 26 years he was senior partner at Mission Psychological Consultants, Inc., a group practice of clinical psychologists, psychiatrists, marital and family therapist, and interns. He is currently Chairman of Physician Well Being at CHOC Hospital @ Mission in Mission Viejo, CA. and adjunct faculty at the California School of Professional Psychology at Alliant International University in San Diego, CA. Dr. Habib is the author of If These Walls Could Talk and has been interviewed by numerous papers, radio and television stations.

HESCAMILLA, HERIBERTO

Heriberto (Beto) Escamilla Morales is originally from Cadereyta Jimenez, Nuevo Leon Mexico. He was raised in Houston Texas until moving with his wife and three children to San Diego in 1984. He received his doctorate in Clinical Psychology from the California School of Professional Psychology-San Diego Campus in 1993. Dr. Escamilla delivered direct clinical services through several community-based organizations and health centers in the San Diego. In addition to professional clinical practice, Dr. Escamilla has taught Psychology and Chicano History classes at San Diego City College and United States University. Dr. Escamilla has a maintained lifelong interest in non-western spiritual and religious traditions including Yoga, Meditation, Prayer and Shamanism. Dr. Escamilla is currently a teaching psychology at United States University, a member of the Center for Integrative Psychology of Alliant University, the National Compadres Network, and as an independent consulting providing technical assistance on cultural competency.

HOWELL, FRANCESCA CIANCIMINO

Francesca Ciancimino Howell received her PhD in Religious Studies from The Open University, UK, and her MPhil in Latin American studies is from the University of Cambridge, Clare Hall, also in the UK. Francesca's research has been involved with relationships between place, nature, and humanity, in various fields and disciplines. She is fluent in Italian and Spanish, and has specialized in performance, ritual, materiality and activism, among other studies. Her most recent research is engaged with the emergence of Paganism and other New Religious Movements in Italy. Prior to carrying out her doctoral research she was on the faculty of Naropa University in Boulder, Colorado. Francesca is currently an Academic Advisor in Spanish and Portuguese at the University of Colorado, Boulder.

KRIPPNER, STANLEY

Biography: Stanley Krippner, Ph.D., is professor of psychology, Saybrook Graduate School and Research Center, San Francisco. He is the former president of the International Association for the Study of Dreams, the Parapsychological Association, the Association for Humanistic Psychology, and two divisions of the American Psychological Association. He is author of Healing tales: The narrative arts in spiritual traditions, Healing stories: The use of narrative in counseling and psychotherapy, and numerous other books and articles.

LAWSON, GARY & ANN

Gary W. Lawson is a Distinguished Professor at Alliant International University's Clinical Psychology program in San Diego. His research interests include: clinical psychology; marriage and family therapy; and chemical dependency. His wife, Ann Lawson, also a Distinguished Professor in the Marriage and Family Therapy program at Alliant University, specializes in family chemical dependency, intergenerational family processes, and family therapy evaluation.

LIGHTHART, LOIS

Lois Lighthart is a native Californian who received her Bachelor's degree in Liberal Arts from Pomona College in1947. She had a brief career teaching primary grades, then later Home Teaching and part-time substitute teaching, K-8. She has been married for 60 years, having two sons and four grandchildren. Lois is now retired at 84 years old. Today her main interest is in Jungian psychology and is an active member in The Friends of Jung society.

LUKOFF, DAVID

Dr. Lukoff is a Professor on the core residential faculty and a licensed psychologist in California whose areas of expertise include treatment of schizophrenia, transpersonal psychotherapy, spiritual issues in clinical practice, and case study methodology. He incorporates many transpersonal approaches in his clinical work including meditation, compassion training, and guided imagery as well as leading groups on spirituality He is author of 70 articles and chapters on spiritual issues and mental health. He has served on the faculties of Harvard, UCLA, Oxnard College, California Institute of Integral Studies, and Saybrook, and been an active workshop presenter providing training for psychologists in spiritual competencies in the U.S., Japan, Mexico, Canada, Brazil, Russia, Romania, Portugal, France, Sweden, Scotland, Ireland, and England.

MARCHI, REGINA

Regina Marchi is Associate Professor in the School of Communication and Information at Rutgers, The State University of New Jersey, where she conducts research on the intersections of media and culture. Before her life in academia, she worked as a journalist in Latin America and the US. She is author of the book DAY OF THE DEAD IN THE USA: THE MIGRATION AND TRANSFORMATION OF A CULTURAL PHENOMENON, which won the James W. Carey Award for Media Research as well as the International Latino Book Award. Regina has published numerous articles in academic and popular publications. An expert in ritual communication and a certified ritual celebrant, Regina creates and facilitates ceremonies of all kinds for family and friends.

McClure, Michael

In the summer of 2008 McClure performed and spoke at The Prague Inernational Writers Festival and in Salerno, Italy for Casa della poesia in Salerno. Michael McClure has long been noted for the popularity of his dynamic poetry performances. At the age of 22 he gave his first poetry reading at the legendary Six Gallery event in San Francisco, where Allen Ginsberg first read Howl. Today McClure is more active than ever, writing and performing his poetry at festivals, and colleges and clubs across the country. "The role model for Jim Morrison," as the Los Angeles Times characterized Michael McClure, has found sources in music from Thelonious Monk and Miles Davis to the composer Terry Riley with whom his poetry readings frequently share a bill. Recently McClure joined with composer Terry Riley to create a CD titled I Like Your Eyes Liberty. The CD explores spontaneous music and voice (working together) expressing the outrageous and mystical in both artists.

Metzner, Ralph

Ralph Metzner, Ph.D. is a recognized pioneer in psychological and cross-cultural studies of consciousness and its transformations. He is a psychotherapist and Professor Emeritus at the California Institute of Integral Studies. He is also the founder and president of the Green Earth Foundation. (www.greenearthfound.org) His books include The Unfolding Self, The Well of Remembrance, Green Psychology, The Expansion of Consciousness, Alchemical Divination and Mind Space and Time

Stream. He is also the editor of collections of essays on ayahuasca and on psilocybin mushrooms.

Mijares, Sharon G.

Dr. Sharon Mijares is an international speaker and author. She has decades of experience in psychology, teaching, leadership and transformation. Her Institutes for Women and Global Change have been given in several nations. She is an international speaker and has enlisted authors representing a variety of cultural perspectives in her first four books. She just completed the fifth.. Dr. Mijares touches many different areas in her work, but each one is focused on improving the human condition.

Overton-Guerra, Shodai Sennin James A.

Some years ago, as the founder of my own martial paradigm MAMBA - Mastering the Art of Mind-Body in Action - I was asked to summarize the essence of my art... Throughout my early childhood and into my middle adolescence my greatest concerns, my ultimate preoccupations focused on overcoming the abject terror and violence that at times defined my existence. Early on in life I realized that the solution to that problem did not reside solely in physical conditioning, technical preparation, or cognitive speculation, for in the face of life-threatening peril if we are without a resilient mental constitution such attributes can quickly uproot and leave us stranded in helplessness and despair... I believe it is for this reason that the real martial arts aim to teach more than just techniques of physical power; they must seek to set the practitioner on a path to the self-empowerment, discovery and improvement that leads beyond an accumulation of information or the memorization of movements - a path which leads to the immutable spirit that derives from mind and body coordinated in harmonious action. This is the Way of MAMBA.

Petry, Judith

Doctor Petry is a Medical Doctor who has retired from the clinical practice of Plastic and Reconstructive Surgery in order to focus her teaching and research on holism in healthcare, alternative systems of healing and the integration of complementary therapies into allopathic medical systems. She functions as a liaison between mainstream health care and complementary therapies for the purpose of optimizing the potential for each individuals healing.

Plotkin, Bill

Bill Plotkin, Ph.D., is a depth psychologist, wilderness guide, and agent of cultural evolution. As founder of southwest Colorado's Animas Valley Institute, he has, since 1980, guided thousands of women and men through nature-based initiatory passages, including a contemporary, Western adaptation of the pan-cultural vision fast. He's also been a research psychologist (studying nonordinary states of consciousness), professor of psychology, rock musician, and whitewater river guide. In 1979, on a solo winter ascent of an Adirondack mountain, Bill experienced a "call to spiritual adventure," leading him to abandon academia in search of his true calling. Bill is the author of Soulcraft: Crossing into the Mysteries of Nature and Psyche, Nature and the Human Soul: Cultivating Wholeness and Community in a Fragmented World, and Wild Mind: A Field Guide to the Human Psyche. He holds a doctorate in psychology from the University of Colorado at Boulder.

Pruginin, Yaron

Dr. Yaron Pruginin, Psy.D., is a licensed psychologist in San Diego, California. He has been helping people with mental illnesses rehabilitate their lives in different settings, including a club-house in Jerusalem, a crisis-house in southern San Diego, a pain management program, and the LGBT counseling services in San Diego. Dr. Pruginin currently focuses on integrating mental health services in primary care pediatric health clinics. He can be reached at Yaronpru@yahoo.com

Reiner, Gail

Gail Reiner is currently working as a family nurse practitioner in au-

tism research funded by the NIH at the Center for Autism Research af-
filiated with UCSD in La Jolla, California. In addition to undergraduate
and graduate degrees in nursing she has a B.A. and M.A. in English literature. She is retired from the School of Nursing faculty at San Diego
State University. She has been funded through private and government
agencies for research and service projects that include a free dental clinic
to provide care to inner city youth, recruiting minority nurses into hos-
pice care, providing nutrition education in Spanish to parents of children
with anemia, and understanding patterns of pain and pain management
in end-of-life patients. She is a 3-year survivor of ovarian cancer.

RIORDAN, PETER

Born in Brooklyn. Grew up in the 'burbs. "Escaped" via the U.S. Navy.
Traveled the east coast of North America from Halifax, Nova Scotia to
Puntas Arenas, Chile and the west from Puntas Arenas to the Aleutian
Islands of Alaska. Deck hand, navigator, skipper. Went back to school after the military, earned an A.A. in graphic arts, am now pursuing my B.A.
in Digital Video Production. I live in the foothills of the local mountains
here in San Diego, California. with my partner of many years Kari Lu and
our four dogs. I write, hike, garden and sculpt. I am looking forward to a
new phase as movie-maker.

ROOST, AIN

Ain Roost is a Clinical and Consulting Psychologist who maintains a
private practice in the San Diego area. He is a Life Member of the Amer-
ican Psychological Association and a Fellow and a past President of the
San Diego Psychological Association. His unique combination of pro-
fessional activities culminated in being honored by his peers with the
Distinguished Contribution to Psychology Award. He is also a former
Olympian, having competed twice as a member of the Canadian Olympic
Team.

ROOST, AMY

Amy Roost worked in the book publishing industry for many years and is currently a freelance writer whose works have been published on numerous popular blogs including MariaShriver.com, ManifsestationYoga.com and PomeradoNews.com. She is also the Executive Director of Silver Age Yoga Community Outreach.

ROSAS, PAULA

I was born in Mexico in 1973 and have enjoyed sharing this world with my parents Leonardo and Marcela and my sister Viviana. I studied Biochemistry and Cell Biology at University of California San Diego, and later obtained a PsyD degree at California School of Professional Psychology, San Diego. I married a wonderful man, Dino, and we have two daughters, Micaela and Silvana, who are a great joy. We all live in Tijuana, Mexico.

RUBANO, JOSEPH

Joseph Rubano is a Biographical Counselor, Spacial Dynamic Movement Educator and poet. He brings 40 years of meditation and inner work, exploring Eastern and Western esoteric traditions, including a strong foundation in Anthroposophy (the teachings of Rudolf Steiner), and years of working with Native American ceremony to his work with individuals, couples and groups. He has been working with the Dyad Communication Process since 1982. And has been offering the True Heart True Mind Enlightenment Intensive and the Desert Solo (Vision Quest) Experience in San Diego and Maine for the past 5 years. He is on the visiting faculty of the Waldorf Institute of Southern California in San Diego and on the faculty of the Biography and Social Art Program at Sunbridge Institute in Chestnut Ridge, New York. He has a private counseling practice in Oceanside, CA where he lives and shares a home with his wife, daughter, and three grandsons.

Saeteng, Issadora

Issadora Saeteng is a health journalism intern completing her fourth year at the University of California, San Diego, where she is majoring in Human Development. Issadora has juvenile onset rheumatic disease, and is planning a career in Counseling Psychology. Issadora works with Dr. Vanessa L. Malcarne, Professor in the Department of Psychology at San Diego State University.

Snyder, Gary

Gary Snyder is an American man of letters. Perhaps best known as a poet, he is also an essayist, lecturer, and environmental activist. He has been described as the "poet laureate of Deep Ecology". Snyder is a winner of a Pulitzer Prize for Poetry.

Solan, Alisha Lenning

Alisha Lenning Solan earned her Ph.D. in Communication Studies from the University of Texas at Austin in 2003. She has more than 10 years of ongoing experience with TranceDance and other ritual work as a participant, assistant, and facilitator. She certified as a TranceDance facilitator in 2007 with Wilbert Alix of the Natale Institute. Dr. Solan has over 15 years of teaching experience at a variety of universities, private schools, and community colleges. She also offers private dissertation and thesis coaching to graduate students in various fields.

Somé, Malidoma

Malidoma Patrice Somé, Ph.D., West African Elder, author and teacher, as representative of his village in Burkina Faso, West Africa, has come to the west to share the ancient wisdom and practices which have supported his people for thousands of years.

Starhawk

Starhawk is one of the most respected voices in modern earth-based spirituality. She is also well-known as a global justice activist and organizer, whose work and writings have inspired many to action. She is the author or coauthor of twelve books, including The Spiral Dance: A Rebirth of the Ancient Religion of the Great Goddess, long considered the essential text for the Neo-Pagan movement, and the now-classic ecotopian novel The Fifth Sacred Thing. Starhawk's newest book is The Empowerment Manual: A Guide for Collaborative Groups, published November 2011, from New Society Publishers

STOLBERG, RON

Ron Stolberg, Ph.D.- Dr. Stolberg is an Associate Professor at Alliant International University in San Diego where he teaches a variety of personality assessment courses. His research interests include assessment in diverse settings, standard of care practices, and social networking in psychology. In his private practice Dr. Stolberg works with suicidal and otherwise high risk teenagers, high caliber professional athletes and on reality TV shows such as Survivor. Dr. Stolberg regularly publishes and presents his research at local and national conferences. He enjoys the outdoors and when not working you are likely to find him on a trail or at the beach. He is married and has two sons.

TELANDER, MARCIE

Marcie is an award-winning writer, psychotherapist, Expressive Arts Therapist, ritualist and festivarian. Marcie is an elder and a founder of the international Cultural Arts and Democracy movement and assists diverse organizations and communities around the country in creating and presenting community unification celebrations. As a bard, poet and storyteller she has led retreats and performed across the country and in Canada, Ireland and Italy. A major part of her practice is working with men and women in developing rites of passage for spiritually creative, life-purpose change. She is the author of the seminal text on the development of personal, intergenerational, story theatre performance--ACTING UP! Marcie has lived, practiced, gardened and celebrated in a cabin on Colorado's East River for 29 years.

WELLAND, CHRISTAURIA

Christauria Welland, Psy.D., is a clinical psychologist in private practice in Solana Beach, CA, with a hospital rehabilitation practice at Scripps Memorial Hospital Encinitas and Paradise Valley Hospital, National City. As a young woman, Christauria dedicated herself to the practice of classical dance (ballet) and modern dance. She then spent 19 years in the Missionaries of Charity of Mother Teresa of Calcutta, living in India, England, Italy, Mexico, and the United States. As a psychologist, she specializes in the treatment of Latino men who are violent to their partners and authored Sin golpes and Healing from violence: Latino men's journey to a new masculinity, as well as several journal articles. She is Adjunct Faculty at Alliant International University in San Diego and teaches at conferences and intensive workshops in the United States, Mexico, Guatemala, and Peru. She expects to continue her international work in healing the wounds of family violence for as long as is humanly possible.

WOLF, FRED ALAN

Fred Alan Wolf is a physicist, writer, and lecturer who earned his Ph.D. in theoretical physics at UCLA in 1963. He continues to write, lecture throughout the world, and conduct research on the relationship of quantum physics to consciousness. He is the National Book Award Winning author of Taking the Quantum Leap. He is a member of the Martin Luther King, Jr. Collegium of Scholars. Former professor of physics at San Diego State University for twelve years, Dr. Wolf lectures, researches, and teaches worldwide. Dr. Wolf has also appeared as the resident physicist on The Discovery Channel's The Know Zone and on many radio talkshows and television shows across the United States and abroad. He took part in the controversial documentary-style films, What the Bleep Do We Know!? and Down the Rabbit Hole.

ZIEGENHORN, LESLIE

Leslie Ziegenhorn, Ph.D. is a Clinical Psychologist. With over 20 years of experience, her study and application of diverse approaches to psychology include the integration of Eastern and Western philosophies. Her formal training in psychology emphasized Cognitive-Behavioral, Developmental, and Jungian perspectives. Since her doctoral education at WSU and postdoctoral fellowship at UCSD, her broad interests have inspired many roles, including psychotherapist, professor, researcher, clinical supervisor, and yoga instructor. Currently, Dr. Ziegenhorn devotes much of her professional time to her private practice in La Jolla, CA and holds faculty positions at UCSD and CSPP/AIU teaching courses such as Human Development, Advanced Developmental Psychopathology, and Working with Dreams in Psychotherapy. Dr. Ziegenhorn volunteers as Faculty Advisor for UCSD's School of Medicine and on the Steering Committee for the Center for Integrative Psychology. She also enjoys travel, hiking, mermaiding, bonfires, and the arts.

ABOUT THE EDITOR

Don Eulert, Ph.D. University of New Mexico, studied post-graduate at the Jung Institute-Zurich. He has served as Fulbright Fellow and lectured abroad on U.S. culture for the State Department. His interest and participation in rituals has taken him from Romania to Kenya, from the Navajo Nation to Thailand. Professor of Integrative Psychology at California School of Professional Psychology, San Diego, his research and teaching include Jung's archetypal psychology; postmodern culture and spirituality; multicultural wisdom traditions; nature-based therapies.

Don's seven books include his poetry, including American haiku, and translations of modern Romanian poetry. He presently coordinates the Center for Integrative Psychology at Alliant International University. For 40 years he has emplaced in the back country of San Diego County on land that was a stop point for the migratory Ipay tribe.

PERMISSIONS

CPSIA information can be obtained at www.ICGtesting.com
Printed in the USA
LVOW13s1809091013

355827LV00001B/1/P